COUi

FACING

MORTALITY

...Cancer Wasn't My Only Obstacle

(Sir) Charles Cary
Foreword by
Tony Browder & Willie Jolley

Trueality Enterprises

Copyright © 2012 by Charles Cary

All rights reserved. No part of this book shall be reproduced
or transmitted in any for or by any means, electronic,
mechanical, magnetic, photographic including photocopying.

Published by:

Trueality Enterprises Publishing

Printed in the United States of America
Published November 2012

Contents

Foreword

I've always been impressed with people who have overcome adversity through strength of character and the masterful use of will power to change the circumstances in their lives. (Sir) Charles Cary is a brother who possesses these qualities and has used these talents to overcome two bouts of cancer while never succumbing to the fear and melancholy that would diminish the spirit of an ordinary man.

Sir Charles Cary is an extraordinary man who exhibited unshakable courage as he faced his own mortality. He has much to share with those of us who can benefit from his profound lessons in healing and there is much we can learn from his experiences. His is a true story of a true survivor.

--Anthony T. Browder, Historian and *Author of Nile Valley Contributions to Civilization* and Director of IKG Cultural resource Center

"Charles Cary is a man on a mission, a mission to help other people to find the untapped strength that they have within, yet far too often do not realize that they have. I have known Charles for a number of years and have always been impressed with his willingness to keep looking deeper and deeper inside himself to find the gifts and abilities that were hidden by situations, circumstances and environment. He grew up in the urban landscape and fell into a pattern that we often see with young people in that environment, drugs and alcohol. Charles struggled with addiction, but looked inside and found strength to overcome it.

He has struggled with relationship issues and eventually divorce, but looked inside and found the strength to survive it and not be bitter. He has struggled with cancer and looked inside and found the strength to look cancer in the eye and make it retreat! He is a man on a mission to help you continue to not just GO through the challenges of life, but to GROW through the challenges of life! This book will help you to do just that! I appreciate Charles Cary for his continued willingness to be transparent and open his life up, in an effort to help others! Bravo Sir Charles, Bravo! I recommend you read this book and then share it with friends, you will be glad you did!"

--Willie Jolley, Best Selling Author of "A Setback For A Comeback" and "An Attitude of Excellence!"

ACKNOWLEDGEMENTS

My friends from ***Frederick Douglas I.S.10*** also known as ***The Dime*** have been an inspiration because the path that I take in this book is a true journey (P.S. 90, P.S.200, and I.S. 10) on how I observed life and how I was becoming influenced. To have connected with some of those friends via *facebook* has been rewarding simply because it reminds me of how it all started (thanks Ricardo Sanchez, Janna Green, and Renee Teenie Wilson).

Norman Thomas High School alumni, I always love you guys (Class of 78). We've come along ways, just like the Virginia Slims commercial back in the day. There are too many names to mention, and so many that might not be remembered all at the same time.

I will say that Eddie Byrd Matthews and I have been on the longest trip, but much love to Renee Teenie Wilson who has also been on that long journey. Additional alumni that are tried and true consist of Billy Taylor, Geoff Hinds, Mike Barlow, Brenda Mack a.k.a. Brenda McLaughlin, Veronica Frazier, Jeffrey Anderson, Adrienne White, Karen Rooks McNair, Debra Knight, Wanda Forden, and trust me the list goes on and on!

We had the greatest high school experience right in the heart of midtown Manhattan. The best think about the relationships that were developed is the fact that almost 40 years later many of us keep in touch several times throughout the year. That includes, baby births, deaths, promotions, books being published and the whole enchilada!

There's a saying that God watches over babies and fools. Well I don't know if I was a baby, a fool, or just a foolish baby, but the Jenkins family, the Hayes family, and the Brown family have been an anchor in my life and I only have God to thank for that. Protectors, overseers, call it what you may, it's all good. All of the family members are best friends and family for life (Carlton

Jenkins, Earl Charles Brown, Larry (Heathcliff) Brown, Walter Hayes)! My life wouldn't have been the same without knowing you.

Learning about personal development and business has been one of the greatest assets in my life. For that I have the teachings of Wayman Hemphill & Bob Crisp for spending so much time in Network Marketing they failed themselves forward into an understanding of the right people equation, and shared it with so many.

Willie Jolley without saying is my greatest hero from a professional standpoint, because he's able to step down from the pedestal that people have placed him on. He's a motivational speaker, he's an entrepreneur, and he's a singer. Most importantly to me he's been a regular
guy, a friend, a brother.

When you travel around the world in your business and you usually only have time to stop and check your watch before the next appointment, but you still make the time for others…that is huge! That's what Willie has done and been for me. Whether it's a phone call, a txt, or an email, he has ALWAYS given me his time.
Fran Briggs, I'd like to thank you for helping me raise awareness about this book set and the importance of it. It's also great having a business alliance that I can learn from.

Reba Barnes, my good cop partner in crime. It's always a pleasure to wheel and deal with you. As long as you remain the good cop, I can be the bad cop ☺.

Jessica Tilles, this project could not have been the same without you. I appreciate all that you've done working. I've learned so much from you and I truly appreciate you.

Lenon, I appreciate ya! Kwan and Enoch…you already know! It takes a special eye to catch the right shot! Photographers 3 The Hard Way!

Monique Medina, A Splash of Moet (little sister), you know I love you and I'm glad that we've finally had a chance to work together. I'm already looking forward to our next project.

Katrina & Nita Bee of Steamy Trails Publishing - Before I knew there was a ST Publishing I knew about Shema Gurls, and I appreciate the reception and the support. Continued Success!

Trueality Enterprises goes into the publishing arena…wow! I never thought this would happen because it wasn't in the plans. If you had asked me about music publishing, I would say yes all day long. I just didn't see this coming!

DEDICATIONS

I dedicate this book to the memory of my brother and to my children. You can do anything that you put your mind to. Never let anyone tell you that you can't, nor let him or her cast doubt upon you. I'm not suggesting that you be difficult with people. I'm simply stating that your limitations should be your own, not dictated by someone's opinion of you, or dictated by what someone thinks you're capable of.

My brother Anthony L. Smith aka Kyleke Allah has meant and will always mean the world to me. Outside of my children, there is none closer to my heart. I hope that in some way brother's spirit lives within me and that his influence has helped shape me.

Mom, you know you are a difference maker and that means the world to me. Many may have prayed for me when I was off track, but your silent tears and prayers were not in vein. I think God spared me of many things because of you and I'm grateful. I love you mother.

Kychel, you were my first born and we've have shared so much I find it simply amazing and a blessing that we've maintain such a wonderful father and daughter relationship. I hope that my granddaughters turn out to be like you and then for sure a legacy will be prominent.

You may not have found what you really want in life yet but it is there within you. Find that quiet still place, so that you can seek it out. Once you find it, never let it go.

Sasha you are the youngest daughter, and I know you are your own person, but never let anyone sway you away from truth. Some truths are hard to bear, but the truth cannot be denied. With God's blessings, you'll have a long and fruitful life ahead of you. Grab hold and never let go. I've always loved you and I always will.

You seem to be taking a serious and mature approach as you've recently met life on life's terms. I hope you keep making positive moves and raise my grandson well!

CJ, I always call you my main man because you are! You're the only son and that doesn't have to be a heavy burden, but just understand this: father's always want their sons to be some big famous person or athlete, but that's not where I'm coming from and I don't want to cast unfair or unreasonable expectations on you. I would just like you to understand that no matter what you do, I love you. I want the best for you, but more importantly you have to want the best for yourself.

This story is about a few different things. I always say that nothing in life is usually singular and everything is the result of a compounded set of circumstances. You will find that this journey is about expectations, about discovery, about acceptance, about love, about failure and about the success of life.

I'm a passionate person and I thank God for allowing me to have a love affair with the creative arts all of my life. In addition, this book will offer *pleasure passion purpose tips*, which are in italics. And poetry that is message oriented.

This story IS NOT written in a chronological order. It's written according to subject matter. I'm hoping you can understand and follow where I'm going because as complex as life is, it can also be complex to revisit it.

The mistakes and mishaps of life happen to many of us. These are mine, but trust me when I say a lesson was learned. There are so many times in life when we feel so uncomfortable, or like we're experiencing such a unique situation and that simply isn't true. Nothing is that unique. We have all made mistakes and have our demons to deal with. I hope you find this to be a good resource.

I'm not special, but I've had a lot of challenges in my life. When I tell people about my drug abuse and troubled past…usually they can't see it. That should be enough to let you know that God still performs miracles

I hope you enjoy **COURAGE FACING MORTALITY …Cancer Wasn't My Only Obstacle.**

Chapter 1

CLAIM IT

Seventeen years ago, I started this project, as I had much to say. With a new keen insight on so many things, I wanted to tell the world. The original title was *A Perfect Life*. I thought, *How clever and how catchy*, and I began writing. I had a new outlook on life. I was going to write about all my girlfriends and everything I learned, getting back at everyone who wronged me. It was going to be a loaded book, but discernment came about me. When I realized what the platform was for, and it didn't matter how big it was, I just needed to learn to respect it and make it count.

I was free from drugs and this sober version of Charles Cary Smith, Sr. was going to share the dos and don'ts of substance abuse, and people were going to listen because after all, Charles was sharing from the bottom of his heart. Forty pages into the project, I suffered from writer's block and the writing ceased.

Several years later, I was inspired to continue my written journey. I added thirty or more pages and was stumped, again, which made me wonder if it was too soon, or if it made sense to want to write my story. After all, I am not a celebrity, who would want to listen to me? Stepping away from the stage was a bit unusual, but as I did that for a few years, there was a void in my life, which caused me to start writing poetry. In fact, I had written so much…it was wild. When I realized how many poems I had written, I couldn't believe it.

This was around the time I was running a home-based business, providing energy and utility services through a third party. During one of the trainings, I heard and met motivational speakers and the appeal to speak really rang home for me. During an annual convention, Les Brown was the keynote speaker, and I was overwhelmed with enthusiasm, and thought to myself, *I can do that*.

After a year of running my business, learning the ins and outs of team building and training, I really felt a kinship with the idea of speaking, training, and motivating, but didn't know the first thing about getting started. So, it was time for the annual convention, and the keynote speaker, once again, was Les Brown. This was confirmation that I needed to follow my heart. After the convention, I started learning about Les Brown, Tony Robbins, Jim Rohn, Brian Tracy, John Maxwell, and all the greats.

I met a speaker from Washington, DC by the name of Willie Jolley. His name should have been Mr. Excited because Willie would just light up a room with enthusiasm the moment he entered and set foot on the stage. Every speaker on the circuit has their own niche. Willie's niche was energy, and the fact that he sang and spoke. In fact, usually he would tell his story of how he was a jazz singer and did all sorts of jingles for almost every major product that you have ever heard.

Willie spoke about his choice, or maybe I should say his motivation, to transition from jazz singer to a motivational speaker. The short version; after doing well at the club, management decided to replace him and his band with a karaoke machine. His first speech led to his next speech, and before he knew it...TADA! He received all sorts of accolades and recognition (it wasn't overnight, but it happened).

On multiple occasions, I would run into this powder keg of motivation named Willie Jolley. However, the one time that really mattered was when he told me, "In order to add credibility to yourself as a speaker, you should have a book." As Arsenio Hall would say, "Things that make you go *hmmm*.

I decided to claim it. I claimed my passion and deep interest of being a motivational speaker. I went on the Internet, read books, ordered books, created a Web site, ordered business cards, and started receiving credentials from my job as a trainer in customer service; I was certified by Homeland Security in Law Enforcement Instruction. It was happening from all sides, but there was no book.

The motivation to finish my book had not appealed to me. The poems were just sitting there and it dawned on me. Publish my book of poems! So I did it. *Poetic Xpressions* was my first published work and I haven't looked back.

When I speak, I inspire. When I train, I inspire. When I sing, on occasion as I do, I try to inspire.

At the time I started writing *Courage Facing Mortality*, I had no idea that I would record four CDs—*Around the Mic w/Sir Charles & Friends*, *Poetic Xpressions* (audio), *Cary's Standards*, and *Cary's Holiday*— is exactly why I know it's important to believe.

Courage Facing Mortality will add value in ways the first book wasn't able to because the subject matter is diverse on various levels.

Claiming your calling is the principle thing. Sometimes, we think we know what we're supposed to do and reality is our purpose may have not been discovered yet. Through *Courage Facing Mortality*, you will find the process in which I discovered my purpose and how you, too, can find yours. I truly believe that if you **Find Your Pleasure, You'll Find Your Passion**, and If You Find Your Passion…*You'll Find Your Purpose!*

Chapter 2

HOW IT STARTED

It all started fifty-some-odd years ago in Washington, DC. I remember living on Irving Street. I was three or four years old. My mother left Washington to work for some wealthy people in Mt. Kisco, New York. She wanted to make some money, so she could get a place and bring all her children together. Mom left us—my sister, my brother and I—with our grandmother. We called my grandmother Mother Dear and my grandfather Father Dear.

My father took my brother and me from Mother Dear's house. Since he wasn't her biological father, he was unable to take my sister, too. I am sure he used aggression and manipulation to get my brother and me, because he wanted Mom back (it was a long shot; can't blame him for trying). He tried to get leverage in any way that he could. He was trying to keep us from Mother, hoping to draw her to him. My brother and I stayed with our father, for as long as he could keep us. Dad knew that Mom wasn't coming back to him. No question.

Mom and Dad's relationship was obviously bad. I wasn't even able to connect the two of them together until I was at least six years old. After serving in the Korean War, Dad worked at the Pentagon as a clerk of some sort. He was married while having a family on the side. I was part of the family on the side. He had the two children with Mom (my brother and I), and three children from his marriage. There were few special times, but DC was home.

Although there were not a lot of fond memories, I remember going to the liquor store off Irving Street with the adults, and the man behind the counter gave the kids bubble gum. That was the highlight of going to the store. I would hope to get a piece of bubble gum or candy. I have forgotten the bulk of activity during those years, but a few things have stuck with me. Hey, I might be dating myself, but I remember the milkman delivering milk, and I still can't understand why people would buy Arco starch and eat it! I also remember how dating was then. My sister Joy's boyfriend, Bip, would come over, and they would sit on opposite sides of the living room, talking. I would peek through the curtains and watch how they interacted. This was how it was done back in the day. I guess you could say it was having company. It would only last for a little while during the early evening.

For better or worse, this is my story and I am going to tell you exactly how it was and how it is. I have brothers and sisters on both sides in my family. On my father's side there was Junior (Paul, Jr.), Lila, Joy, and I vaguely remember someone else (I think her name was Tiny), but it was so long ago. Their mother was Mary who I believe was legally married to Dad. Mom had Cecelia, Tony, me, and Monique. Leon was Cecelia's father, but Monique's father was Pete, and my brother and I have the same parents. To be honest, I felt honored to have brothers and sisters and I have never spoken to them or looked at them as step- or half-sisters and brothers. I was a kid full of love and I loved the idea of having siblings and being a sibling. Even Angie, who is technically my stepsister, is my sister period. She and Monique have the same father (Pete).

I was a constant thinker, even as a young child. The mental voice was so active, not knowing those were thoughts that could lead to actions and expression. I had very little awareness as a child, until my stepfather told me, one day, to be observant. Then and only then did the wheels slowly start turning. I seemed to have questioned everything. What people didn't understand about me was that I was truly seeking understanding—what something was, how it worked, why it existed—I honestly wanted to know. As a child, many adults viewed this as back talk, or my being a smart-ass, or trying to be grown. I have a brain and I thrive off understanding, especially if I am interested.

I was so intimidated when I found my new home. New York, New York—so nice they named it twice! There was a tremendous difference coming to New York from Washington, DC. I had never seen a building that was over three stories tall. I had an Afro going on, and it was only 1964. People wore Afros, but it wasn't "the style," at least not yet. New York was really something to me. It was an all-out culture shock. Kids all over the place, walking, running, riding bikes, jumping rope, spinning tops, and yo-yo's. I remember wanting to look out the window and when I did, there were bars on it. You had to stick your hand through the gate to open the window just to get some air. We lived in a fifth floor walkup, in the back of the building. Living in an apartment building wasn't anything like a house. There was a stoop in New York, but a porch in DC, bars and gates seemed to be all over New York, but I never noticed anything like that in DC.

I would soon share and experience life in a way that seemed unreal to me. One of my most traumatic experiences was when our apartment was robbed. I was all of six or maybe seven years old. I had arrived home from school to find that our apartment was in serious disarray. My first thought was that my mom, brother, or sister was cleaning up, and they had not yet finished. However, realizing I was home alone, and the way the apartment was ransacked, scared me. So I hid under the bed. After a few minutes, I crawled from under the bed, stepped out of our apartment and into the hallway. When I heard someone coming up the stairs, and realized it wasn't anyone from the family, I went back into the apartment, closed the front door and got under the bed again. I wanted to be brave, yet things didn't seem to add up in my young mind.

It started feeling spooky, so I came out from under the bed and opened the front door. However, this time, I kept it opened, and it was only a matter of minutes when I heard my brother coming up the stairs. By the time Mom came home, it was obvious we'd been robbed. The thieves came in the window from the

roof. They didn't bother any items that belonged to me; they only

took household items and clothes that belonged to my stepfather.

The police arrived to take a report, and that was an experience for

me. I kept looking for their gun while they were talking to my

momma. She was crying, and clothes were strewn all over the

place. Pete, my stepfather, thought that in some way it was my

brother's fault. Tony always seemed to be at fault, even by default.

Chapter 3

REFLECTION

I had relatives who resembled celebrities. I had an uncle who resembled Sugar Ray Robinson, and a cousin named Rodney, who resembled Michael Jackson. I don't know about the talents, attributes, or skills from Dad's side of the family. I think most of them did the traditional thing—got a job and worked—except for the gambling and drinking. That side of the family was wild. They would come together on a Friday or Saturday and start upstairs just talking. There were times when talking turned into arm wrestling and trash talking, then grown men wrestling on the floor, tumbling over each other, trying to see who could pin the other one or who could out-do who. It was like the WWF, and I had a front-row seat. Aunt Virginia would be screaming at them because they would knock over lamps, break dining room tables; break up any furniture that was in the way.

When it comes to talent and positive attributes, my mother was a star. She sang very well as a youngster, as I have been told. She, along with her siblings, had a group in church. They were The Brown Singers, singing at various church services. I don't think Mom had aspirations of being a professional singer, but she had the talent to sing and that is a fact. Many years later, my uncle sang with a group called The True Tones. For thirty years, he sang and wrote songs with them. At first, they were the Dynamic True

Tones, and then they were The Sensational True Tones and, finally, The Amazing True Tones.

In the mid-sixties, The Sensational True Tones shared billing with many groups such as the Gospel Keynotes, The Violinaires and The Mighty Clouds of Joy. They were definitely just as good in their own right. They were very hot on the local gospel circuit and recorded seven or eight albums with numerous 45s. My cousin, Elder Joseph Jackson, also known to the family as Jo-Jo, played with the True Tones for a while. Jo-Jo plays guitar, keyboards and sings up a storm. He really gets down on that guitar (playing with his teeth and all that). He recorded with my uncle's group a few years back before my uncle got sick and stopped singing. Elder Jackson records his own albums these days. His sister, Geraldine, used to whip the drums something terrible. In fact, all of my aunt's children can go. Gregory, Geraldine, Elder Jackson, I don't know about cousin baby sis, or my cousin Linda, but the others get down.

We traveled back to DC for family vacations. Each time we would visit Sharon Baptist Church with Mother Dear and Father Dear or my aunt's church. I looked forward to hearing the music at Aunt Lois's church; hearing her or a cousin singing would be a highlight for me. I guess I was looking for confirmation, because of the yearning burning inside of me. Those early exposures to music let me know that there was something special that my family had within. I would later learn the liberation of tapping into it. My music heroes were James Brown, The Motown Sound (The Supremes, The Temptations, and especially Michael Jackson and Jermaine Jackson) and Earth Wind & Fire. That era was most educational for me. My first personal experiences with music and performing took place when I was very young. Like most kids, I started singing with the radio and then to 45s and LPs. I was beating on empty oatmeal boxes and the like. While in school, the thought of being in band class was fascinating to me.

As a kid, my lungs (wind) were good; I played the clarinet from sixth to eighth grade. I was so happy when I was given an opportunity to take my instrument home. Instead of totally focusing on the sheet music that I was given in school, I immediately started trying to play any tune that I had ever heard on the radio. I was so excited about playing an instrument, that when it was time to attend high school, I decided to audition for the famous High School of Music & Arts in Harlem. At that time, I wasn't a good musician. The kids who auditioned, and were accepted, were exceptional musicians, singers, and dancers. I always tried to take the short cut in music class. I would play the easy arrangements, not wanting to challenge myself.

Because of my family's musical background, it was hurtful when my music teacher told me days before my audition that I wasn't as good of a musician as I should be. When I think about it, I am glad he expressed his feelings to me. However, at that time, it was a shot of reality that I wasn't ready to hear.

On the audition, I was extremely nervous. I got dry mouth and started my piece at least twice. The judges knew I wasn't an A student in musicianship. A few years later, I discovered my singing voice and started singing with a local church, and then on to another church choir and ensemble.

We had several childhood friends who didn't make it out of childhood. Some overdosed, went to jail or juvenile homes, were killed in car accidents or killed by riding on the back of buses. Jumping on the back of a bus was popular in the early '70s. Kids would jump on the back of the bus, not have to pay a fare and show off in the process, but the risk of being killed was a major deterrent for me. It is very sad when you think of it. They didn't have a chance to grow up. I walked through those years very carefully. Other difficulties I had were having my fresh young heart broken. I couldn't understand why girls played so many darn games. I understood very little at that time.

My brother ran away from home often. I didn't understand why he did this nor did I understand why my mother and father were not together. There were so many unanswered questions…so many unsure feelings. Maybe that was why I got in trouble for asking questions. I really didn't comprehend what was happening to my family around me, but it was important for me to grasp these things.

How we've changed is a big deal and then again it isn't. Today women talk and talk, and in many cases they play different games—I don't know what you're talking about, and the "I never said that" game. It's amazing how we go through life and various experiences, and we still don't act like we know. We live life as if its a game. Then when things don't go the way we want we're surprised, and then we repeat the process. Humans are supposed to be the most intelligent beings on the planet. Go figure. Relationships seem to be the most complicated, yet the easiest thing to have in life, but we know how to mess them up real good.

During the late '80s, I went on casting calls and various auditions around New York City, including the famous Apollo Theatre. I played all over the city in bands, or by doing track dates (music performed on CDs or cassette dates). I sat home and watched *The Jacksons: An American Dream* several years after it aired. There had been a lot of talk about Michael Jackson and his eccentric behavior, so the networks were cashing in on everything they could. As I watched the movie, I became very emotional, and it made me reflect on how my life wasn't always peachy. So many moments were filled with pain and growth, so I related to their story.

One thing about music is that she has always been true to me. Between the ages of fourteen and thirty, I performed throughout the northeastern seaboard before thousands of people. *Star Search* told me my sound was too urban. It was only natural that I would audition at the Apollo. When auditioning for the

Apollo, all performers had to take a number. I was excited. I met a guy on line while I was waiting. His name was Mike. We decided to perform together. The best song I could think of was *There's Nothing Better Than Love* by Luther Vandross and Gregory Hines. We finally got to the stage, and it was time to get busy. As the song started, I did my part. When Mike was supposed to start singing his part, he blanked out and forgot the words. The judges shifted and excused us. I knew immediately I had blown my chance.

My youngest sister lives in New York and from time to time, she would hang around with some of the big female names in rap. I know lil' sis is talented, but our talents are always channeled through us at various times, depending on what stage of life we are in. I wanted to share more of my musical knowledge with my little sister, but she was so damn bad when she was young, so I just focused on myself. The good thing is that she tapped into her creative talents without much encouragement.

It is said that opportunity only comes once, maybe twice, within your lifetime. I believe that, but, for some reason, I also believe I am different. With all I am made of, and with all I have done and heard, I can do things that other people may not be able to do. The funny thing is I don't think I am so much more talented than anyone else is, but I just have the feeling within me that if you believe, it can happen. That carries a lot of weight, especially if you are willing to speak it into fruition. Life and death is in the

power of the tongue!

Chapter 4

THE BIG APPLE

My parents took me shopping to prepare me for the first grade, and I caught a crook in my neck from staring up at all the tall buildings. Before school started, I needed to get a whole lot of fine-tuning. My sister, Cecelia, taught me how to tell time. She also worked with me on the alphabets. My soon-to-be stepfather taught me a few basics about math, and my mother taught me my address and telephone number. I attended P.S. 90 around the corner from where we lived.

It was truly a culture shock, moving from DC to New York. I didn't know it then, but peer pressure directed me and I was almost a slave to it. I was influenced by the ways of the street. I didn't get off to a great start, but I guess bad is bad. At a young age, I didn't know how to direct myself. I would get into little stuff. I picked a fight with a fat kid named Sammy while in the second grade. The kid wore eyeglasses. I would put thumbtacks in kids' chairs. I tried to manipulate another kid while in the second grade, but it didn't work out too well. Jeffrey Bradley came to school early one day and I tried to rough him up by talking bad, and trying to see if I could scare him. He was ready. He told me "Let's fight," and I said, "Okay," but he put me in a chokehold, and out of frustration, because I couldn't break my way out, it made me back down.

Meanwhile, my brother was beating up kids and teachers in predominantly white schools in Queens. He came home late almost every day. Sneaking around with girls was one of his favorite past times. Me personally, I am a homebody at heart. I didn't need to do a lot because I knew how to entertain myself, but when we first moved to New York, part of me was curious about the outside world. I had to learn the neighborhood (although I knew I wasn't very confident in my new surroundings). I embarked on some local shopping, so that I would know my way around. I would encourage my mother to send me, because I needed that sense of confidence. Other kids knew the area and were very streetwise. Eventually, I started to do major shopping at the supermarket. I would have a list, do comparative shopping, use coupons and bring back the correct change. I even got mugged a couple of times (induction into the real world).

From pictures I have seen and stories told to me by other relatives, my dad, Paul, was a good-looking and a very well-dressed man. Dad didn't get along with my grandparents. I guess there were many reasons. Dad was an overly jealous man, a womanizer and consumed alcohol. Early, I imagine things were good between Mom and Dad. As they had gotten to know each other, they found out the undesirable traits of one another. My father's jealousy and drinking only got worse, and Mom's religious and disciplined lifestyle was less accepting of that. He would want to show Mom off, because he knew he had a fine catch. Dad would show off and showcase Mom's vocal talents, asking her to sing in front of his friends and being very disappointed if she didn't honor his request. I think Dad was physical with Mom at times. He was a decent man; he just bit off more than he could chew from time to time.

Unfortunately, he also was an alcoholic. When he couldn't afford the better-quality alcohol, he extended himself to the drink of the next level. Wine was one of his main substitutes, as far as I can remember. His side of the family seemed to get together daily to drink, play cards, gamble—numbers, etc.—or wrestle in the living room.

I can remember as far back as two or three years old just watching grown people; watching their ways and mannerisms. It was quite interesting, songs of the '50s and '60s setting the tone. The kids were put to bed, so the grownups could party. I would peek through the curtains to see what they were doing. They would be dancing real close on songs like *Don't Mess with Bill*. I was always checking something out. There were folks running in and out of the house, playing numbers or hustling up money for a bottle of liquor or cigarettes. Gambling was an everyday event. Those were the times, and that is just the way it was.

When I was four years old, my brother, while riding his bike in a major intersection in DC, was hit by a car. I didn't see it, but I heard the adults talking about it. I was crying and in my own little world. I was so upset, because my brother was everything to me. I will never forget the feelings and the loneliness. After my brother recovered from the accident, he ran away. It seemed as if my brother was a piece to the puzzle in my life that I learned so much from. He was always getting into trouble. He was so disobedient. He was always running away from home. He would leave DC and go to New York; he would get in trouble for so much. I love my brother tremendously. Words can't express the sorrow I feel for his absence.

It was a crucial time for me. One I will always treasure for the rest of my life. It was one of the first transitions I would acknowledge. I really had forgotten the faces of my mother and sister, but I would know them when I saw them. It was the summer of 1964. Dad was taking me to the liquor store, which I thought was great, but little did I know that the moment I set my foot out the door that I would be on my way to New York City.

I saw my brother walking down the street with my mother and sister. I loved my brother so much I wondered at times if I loved him more than I loved Mom. He was the only person I had been around consistently then. Daddy and I hit the street and before my eyes was my brother, the most precious sight I could have the pleasure of beholding. He was walking with my mother and sister Cecelia, and they were coming to get me. BAM! I took off like a rocket. I jumped right into my brother's arms, calling his name repeatedly. Daddy was very sad about this, because he knew

Momma was coming to take me away. I just felt it in my heart. We left and went to see my grandmother over on 14th Street.

The transition wasn't so smooth for me. When I lived in Washington, all I did was play. Now it was time to learn and prepare for life. I was a quiet kid who got along with the others, but I was a true introvert. I slowly learned, but surely. I was trying to fit in. My brother was aggressive and seemingly troubled. I don't like describing him that way, but I find I gravitate to the description, because it is a given. Cecelia was doing well in school and after graduating high school; she would relocate back to DC.

On the way to New York, I was so excited I stood up in the car for the entire four-hour drive. I didn't know what to think about the big city. Everything was so big and so tall and intimidating. Where I came from, the tallest building was about three stories high. The church that I would attend was right downstairs—7th Avenue Mennonite. I would spend a number of years in that church, and it touched a number of young people in the community.

The Mennonites had churches in all five boroughs. Collectively, there was a core of Mennonites in Pennsylvania. The location that was considered the Headquarters was in Lancaster, Pennsylvania. Lancaster seemed to be one of the last places resembling the old country, with Quakers and many people living off their land. Collectively the churches pooled their monies to purchase some land many, many years ago with the intention of having outreach groups, as well as seminars.

This area was called Camp Deer Park located in Deer park, New York. It was a well-groomed program. Certain age groups were scheduled to attend camp at the same time, bringing different neighborhoods together. There was also wilderness camp where we slept out in the woods and learned the ways of nature. If you were really too young, then you went to the Fresh Air Fund. I guess I was lucky, because I could do both. Every year, I went to the Fresh Air Fund, and when I was old enough I went to Camp Deer Park, and I would cry every year when it was time to go to camp.

Camp was a real growing experience for me. Being a kid could be rough, but overall I would say it was great. I learned about different types of people. I learned about whites, blacks, Amish, Baptist, prejudice and everything. Those experiences really helped to mold my life. I learned about house manners; how each set of family values can be entirely different. People can be from the same state or city, and have entirely different mannerisms and lifestyles. As a child, I remember certain situations that were not pleasant and some things were just really bad.

Once, I embarrassed myself at the dinner table, because I thought it was impolite to make a sandwich at the dinner table. When I was at the Fresh Air Fund, staying with a Mennonite family (The Herrs), I smacked a sandwich out of Neven's hand. I didn't know; I just thought that it was something you didn't do at dinner. While living in Harlem as a youngster, my cousin and I almost burned down an apartment building. I don't remember the outcome of the situation, but I learned a lot about getting out of things at an early age.

I wonder was it because of the times or was it just a phase? I do feel that I have learned a lot over the years in regards to lying, drug use, getting over, stealing and all of those combined negative traits. What goes around definitely seems to come around in one way or another.

From the mid-sixties to mid- eighties, I attended church regularly and participated in various programs and recitals.. I still have a Bible that was given to me from the Mennonite Church about forty years ago. Initially, going to church was odd for me. I wasn't used to doing anything as a toddler. There was no preparation for kindergarten or primary school. When my mother came to get me from my father, I was sort of in shock. Now, I had to learn my address and all sorts of things. Attending church was a bit much for me. I didn't have the attention span for it. It was good for me. It was my foundation. After all I have experienced as a young adult, the upbringing and the church showed me what I should and should not be doing.

One season I played basketball on the church team. We had green and white jerseys and lost every game. Since I was the tallest of all the boys, my position was center. We played against the inner-city teams in our division, and they pounded us. There were games against Resurrection and Minisink, and we were demolished. I scored in three out of twelve games (ten total points during the season). All of my baskets were made by chance. My brother was locked down on Rikers Island when I played on the church team. Before he went to jail, he played on the church team also, with the older boys. He did a lot better than I could ever do. I found out years later that when I wrote letters to my brother in jail, it made him cry. I wanted my brother to be a big part of my life.

These were special times, lonely times and curious times. I don't know if I realized that we were poor. My mom and stepfather always seemed to do what was right. At least that was what they told us, and that was how it appeared. We always had food, clothing and a place to stay. The basics helped to keep us going and I was content with a few GI Joe's and a black and white TV.

Can you believe I was circumcised at seventeen years old? What an experience. I will not go into what happened, but I had to have the procedure to prevent infection. The day of the procedure, I was rolled into the operating room. The doctor began pouring this cold solution over my penis. When I say cold, it was very cold. The nurse was walking around, back and forth. She stopped and asked me if I would like to listen to some music. I asked her to put on WBLS 107.5. That was the station I listened to. So we have Nurse Smiley Face walking around, cold solution between my legs and me not knowing what to expect. You talking about somebody being nervous, that was no joke. I had never had an overnight stay in the hospital prior to that. My dad had taken me to get circumcised when I was much younger, but I was crying so much and so hard he came back to get me that same day. The doctor started to cut me, and he wanted to know if I could feel it. I told him I could; he put more solution on me and started the surgery. I felt like a rubber band being cut.

The stitching started immediately after the foreskin was removed. The foreskin was placed into a glass jar; I caught a glimpse of it floating around. The nurse came back in and said, "It's the same size." I thought that chick was loony. Anytime I got an erection, it hurt like a mug. Knowing that my girl was coming for a visit took a lot of concentration. I had to think of ice cream, cold water, and winter, whatever it took, so there was no erection. The doctors told me that I would require at least eight-weeks to heal.

After the eight-weeks I did what the doctor told me, I soaked in the hottest water I could stand and took off all the gauze wrapped around the incision. I was so anxious, but I was scared because I knew it was going to hurt. I was scared to put my seventeen-year-old butt in that water, but I did it. Gingerly, layer-by-layer, I peeled off the gauze in the hot water. All I could think about was going to the doctor to get his blessing and calling up my girlfriend to be reacquainted.

I went to the doctor and he was so upset with me. I didn't understand what the problem was with that whacko.

"I told you to take off the gauze," he said.

"I did," I replied.

"There is still one layer left. Go home and take off the gauze the same way I told you before."

My heart sunk. I couldn't believe it. The layer of gauze was discolored so much that I thought it was my skin. I wanted to yank it off just like they do in the movies when people have their mouths taped up. When I removed the final layer, I couldn't wait to have sex. That is no lie.

Chapter 5

PUNISHMENTS

Being raised with discipline is very important for a child. For me, it was a shock. I wasn't used to anyone talking loud to me, or hitting me. After being in New York for about a year or so, I learned a very discomforting phrase that Pete would repeat with vengeance and furious anger! He would threaten, "I'll bust your ass wide open." Just the thought of it was scary. However, the education was just starting. I went to the school of Hard Knocks and Bricks University. One time, in particular, I will never forget it. I was given a list to pick up a few things from different stores. I returned home asking for more money and my parents couldn't understand why I needed more. I had stashed a five-dollar-bill in my back pocket for a different item and had forgotten about it. When I returned from a successful store run, my parents wanted to know what happened to the money, and why I needed more, and I really didn't know what to say. I was told to empty my pockets and the five-dollar-bill fell out; I was shocked. I was beaten until I admitted I was trying to steal it, although I wasn't trying to steal. Situations like this taught me about truth, honesty, right and wrong, good and bad, and I learned this lesson early on in life. Yet, I still continued to repeatedly make unwise decisions.

Most holidays were cool as far as I can remember. There were the cookouts, trips to the park, and occasionally there would be some event, probably free that we would attend. Christmas was always pretty hot. I was the king of action figures. I had army men, cowboys and Indians and all this other stuff. My prize possessions were the twelve-inch action figures, such as GI Joe and all of his enlisted friends in the service, and Johnny West and his wife Jane (The Best of the West); I had all the equipment and accessories. Yeah, Christmases were nice.

I didn't have the latest fashions. I wore Skips, before I graduated to PF Flyers (tennis shoes), which I soon traded for a pair of Chuck Taylor's, and then finally a pair of PRO-Keds. Who cared if by the time that acquisition went down the new thing was Super PRO-Keds? I wore cotton slacks and shirts while my friends wore double knits and polyester shirts. I felt like I was always behind everybody, but I did get my chance. I learned about fitting in. I realized how important it was to have the latest, to be cool, to look hip. Eventually, I rose to higher ranks. I also understood that it was better to have something than nothing at all.

As I got older, my parents bought me clothes from Barney's New York, but I was only allowed to wear them on Sundays, a special occasion, or when I had permission. The point was you had to learn what acceptance was and live with it. My brother, Tony, and I used to get moderate to severe beatings as punishment when we did something wrong. It was usually with a belt or a strap of some type. I suppose Pete had beaten us the way he did because that was how he was disciplined, or there was just some aggression he felt needed to be worked out on our asses. There was probably a combination of a bunch of stuff going on in his head. In today's society, that type of ass whipping would be labeled abuse, but then it was called tough love. Coming from a person with a history of problems with their nerves, I doubt if he should have been the one to try to keep us in line. I wanted to follow Tony's lead, and run away from home, but had no place to go.

When we got into trouble or did something that was considered unacceptable, there were several options to consider for punishment—no going outside, no TV, no company, no sleepovers, and restrictions for two weeks or from one report card to another. These were serious punishments. Kids today should endure these types of corrective behaviors. It's sad to say, but today's kids would probably murder their parents if they were subjected to this type of treatment. There was one incident where my parents should have shared the blame with me, but they didn't. They left me home alone while they went out to a party, and I played with matches. When they got home, the smell of sulfur consumed the house. Bored with being home alone, I built stick houses and set them on fire, so I could see the chain reaction. Of course, my parents didn't see it my way, so they let my hind part take all the blame. The part that hurt worse was that Mom gave me that thrashing. She never hit us, well not me.

Tony and I discussed killing Pete several times. Although I didn't like the way he disciplined us, I knew killing him would be a sin. I was scared and knew the police would get involved. However, Tony didn't care; we needed to get him. As an adult, after my brother had long disappeared, I thought about killing him, too, because of how he was manipulating my mother and her love for him.

Tony hated Pete for the way he disciplined us, and because he appeared to be white. As kids, we didn't understand that he was mixed with Spanish blood and probably some other ethnicity. The kids in my class used to tease me, saying I was Puerto Rican, because they saw my stepfather, and because I spit between my teeth. That used to bother me. I didn't know what a Puerto Rican was. Pete used to say, "I am light, not white." I think the other kids in the neighborhood used to tease my brother about it. I got my share of being teased also. I had no clue what they were talking about. What's a Puerto Rican?

As for the discipline, it came to a point where Tony wouldn't cry if he had gotten a beating. He told me not to cry. We broke it down to a science. Did it really hurt? Yeah. Did it hurt enough to make us cry or was it just the shock of being hit? It was definitely the shock of being hit. That startling feeling, okay I get it. From that point on, I would never cry again—not from a beating or anything else imaginable—at least, not for a long time. It worked, too, because Pete noticed. He said, "You are being like your brother, huh?" I think it really bothered Pete that we

refused to cry. Soon afterwards, the beatings subsided. What was

the use? If you can't see your prisoner suffer, why punish them?

After that, he threatened to punch us. I believe he hit Tony

a couple of times, and again Tony ran away from home. How

should things have been handled? Whose fault is it? Does it matter

now? Dare I write about it? Sometimes I get pissed just thinking

about it and sometimes I feel pain. Meanwhile, Tony was a regular

"run away." He had already started his bad-boy lifestyle and I

guess I was trying to toughen myself up by being unruly. Most

kids have a fresh mouth, occasionally. I was never the type that

would talk about people or talk about other kids' mothers. I didn't

have the knack with words or know-how to run the dozens (we

used to call it snapping on each other). What I did was stay quiet

most of the time to learn.

Punishments are necessary, but how you go about it is the

key. Growing up I experienced some stiff punishments. Not all of

which were needed, but I wasn't broken. From the punishments, I

have learned that there is more than one way to handle a situation.

I have also decided that I will not raise my children the same way,

just because that was how I was raised.

Chapter 6
WHO WAS I?

I was the type of kid who could take a dollar, go to the movies, get my popcorn, candy, and soda and be content all day. I didn't even need company. I would go to the movies by myself in a heartbeat. Even when I learned slang, it didn't seem to be my preference or style. I knew how to go there, but it wasn't important. It seemed unnatural coming from me. Whenever I tried to sound hip, it would be one or two words that sounded very catchy. Anything beyond that, and I would be taking a chance at putting myself out there. I think the worst thing I did in those early years was play hooky. I played hooky for two weeks, and I was scared to death, too. I just knew I was going to be caught, but it never happened. I veered away from the school. I went to the park. I also played with younger kids. I came home at the end of the school day just like everything was all right.

It was around Easter, and a postcard came home from school. Mom decided to read it when we returned from Easter clothes shopping. There was a girl in our class by the name of Betty, and all the boys teased her until one day she cried. Our principal, Mr. Sellers, liked Betty. The way she was crying, you would have thought somebody literally kicked the crap out of her. I was scared to death. I never said much to her, but I did say something and one of the other boys was quick to remind me that I was involved. I was so scared I refused to go back to school,

because we were going to be in trouble by Mr. Sellers.

Meanwhile, Momma and Pete were picking out my clothes

at the store. I was scared because I had not been to school. I didn't

have a note. I simply didn't know what to do. The whole time my

parents were trying to dress me up in the store, I didn't want to ask

for a thing. I knew I wasn't worthy. I also knew when Pete found

out he would probably want to *bust my ass wide open,* as he would

eloquently state it. When we got home and they read that postcard,

saying that your child hasn't been to school for two weeks, I got

sick all over. I started throwing up. That was how scared I was. I

froze up right on the spot. I wanted to say, "It was all because this

girl named Betty threatened to tell the principal that all of the boys

in the class were teasing her." My mind was racing a mile a

minute. I didn't know how to respond. Then I tried to act like I

didn't know what Mom was talking about.

A tall dark-skinned man, Mr. Sellers was strict. I was easily

spooked. I didn't like getting beatings, and I didn't like getting in

trouble. I never got in trouble in school before. Those were the

days of corporal punishment, teachers, and neighbors correcting

kids freely. Pete's mother thought it was funny. She prevented me

from getting a beating. I think I was on punishment for a few

weeks. I guess that was one experience that spooked me. They

were so angry with me. If you think about it, anything could have

happened to a seven-year-old kid playing hooky for that length of

time. The primary school years were an education, and I am not
talking academics.

I remember another time when Tony and I were going to
Bear Mountain, and he couldn't find his keys. We looked all over
the house and still no keys. Tony was really related to something
called *TROUBLE,* so knowing him he probably hid his keys, so
that they wouldn't make noise as he snuck in the house the night
before. I suggested we pray to God, and He would help us. He got
real angry and cursed God. We were supposed to meet the buses at
8:00 am. I prayed anyway. I must have been about eight years old.
The moment my prayer ended, I walked down the hall into the
living room. Tony continued looking all over. I stood in the
hallway, and turned to my right and looked in the living room.
BINGO, there they were! The keys were dangling from the
magazine rack. I had looked before and didn't see them. I yelled
out, "I found them." He looked at me with such frustration and
anger; he simply didn't know how to respond; all he could say was
"Come on, let's go!" I have never really cried about my brother's
disappearance. I feel that I will see him one day before I die.

One of my cousins would call me a gangster because I
refused to rat on the other kids. When something went wrong, the
adults would probe me for information—I never budged. I would
tell exactly what they wanted to know, nothing more. If they asked
the wrong question, oh well. I tried to get along with people. I
wasn't the fighter, but I met the bully of the school. It seemed like

he could fight, play sports, had the girls and everything. He really was a nice guy who just loved having control and getting people to do what he wanted. Alphonso Carter was his name. He was short, a nice dresser and a cool kid. I never told anyone that Carter was trying to have all the second grade boys under his thumb. One day, Tony found out about Carter. Carter would manipulate or finesse anyone into doing what he wanted. If that didn't work, he would beat them up.

He never beat me up, but I was definitely unsure of myself. One day, Tony told me how to stand up for myself and how important it was for me to protect myself. I wasn't taking this information seriously. He asked me if I was scared of anybody and the only person I could think of was Carter. He was so mad at me for not telling him what was going on. He insisted that I never be afraid of anyone and that I stand up for myself. One day, he met me after school and spoke to Carter. From that day on, I guess Carter and I were supposed to be lifelong friends—it never happened. In most situations like that I probably should have been Carter's partner in crime, but I wasn't that type of kid.

Carter continued to bully the other kids, but he didn't bother me. Wanting to belong put me in a position where I have felt alone or pressured at various times in life. My next challenges would be worst. . Once in junior high school, I was having a bad day, and this boy said something to me that I didn't like. I recall saying to him "Your mother," and I thought it was over. He came behind me and asked me what I said. I felt vindicated, initially, because after my initial response he didn't say anything else. I let my guard down and when he approached me in the locker room he had me. He asked me again "What did you say?" I was unsure how to answer. He put his hands up and we started swinging. A crowd quickly gathered and I got nervous. My friends were all there, and I expected someone to break it up.

The fight should not have lasted as long as it did. He caught me with a couple of good shots before tripping over something. By then, with all the attention, I was scared. He had me cornered. He punched me in the face and, as soon as his fist hit my face, I yanked my head back to get out of the way and it ricocheted into a cement wall. I was knocked out for about five or ten seconds. I was too embarrassed to tell anyone that didn't already know, and I learned a valuable lesson: STAY TRUE TO SELF. It wasn't like me to talk about somebody or his or her mother, so I should not have said what I said. I should not let myself go there. I've always been that way. That same kid attended the same high school I attended. He got into a fight with a girl who also went to junior high school with us. I think he was expelled from school. He was a bad seed or considered as such. I guess if I had beaten him that day in the locker room, things *may have* turned out much different for me and definitely to him.

Chapter 7

FATHER LOVE

In 1968, my biological dad was murdered. From what I can remember about his death, he had a boarder staying at his place. This boarder was behind on his rent payments. My dad just happened to come upstairs from the basement, where the rest of the family and friends were partying and gambling. He approached the boarder about being behind in his rent, and the boarder wasn't trying to hear it. There was an exchange of words between the two men. Dad tried to stop him from going to the room he was renting, and the boarder stabbed him in the liver. My father fell to the floor and bled to death.

The boarder was apprehended, but I don't remember how long he was incarcerated, or any of the details relating to the case. It was a very cold November, and Tony and I took a Trailways bus from New York to Washington, DC for the wake and funeral. As usual, I got sick on the bus. Motion sickness was something my young body couldn't tolerate.

Daddy had a military funeral, because he was a veteran from the Korean War or Conflict. The funeral had very little impact on me, because of my age. I didn't realize at the time it meant I would never see my dad again. He was laid out in a nice brown suit, and I also remember seeing lots of family members. I had a picture of Dad in his casket for the longest. I think all I have now are a few cuff links, and maybe a tie clip.

My father's death upset Tony tremendously, because he would run away from home to escape Pete. I imagine that although my dad wasn't a fool, he knew he lost my mom to Pete. Although it was probably his own fault from years of compounded conflict and alcoholism, my father gave my mother away to the next relationship opportunity that would present itself to her.

After Daddy's death, Tony would run away from home to stay with friends. Running away was probably a small or temporary victory for him, but Daddy's death spelled final in so many ways outside of the obvious. The relationship between Tony and Pete took a long time before it became tolerable. .

I missed the actual relationship with my biological father. I didn't get a chance to toss a ball back and forth with him, ask him some of those hard questions about life, or talk to him about life with my mom back in the day. It would have been interesting to know how his life was as a boy. There are all sorts of questions I would have loved to have known the answers to. I once heard a message from TD Jakes on a CD I bought. Bishop Jakes said that a boy needs his father, and then he went on to say that he's learned a man needs his father, too.

Now I know that I am emotional, but the paternal instincts, feelings, and emotions are real. Just like a mother's instincts kick in, so do mine. I love my children deeply, and I constantly advocate they know each other, ask each other questions; have a relationship outside of me. It was made clear to them that I will not always be around, and no matter who their mother is they are linked as siblings.

When I was away from my first born, I felt her need for my nurturing. Because the pain within me was so great, and I was immature, I didn't know how to handle it. However, I am glad that I have a full relationship with my daughter. We talk like old friends who have not seen each other in ages. Sometimes, we chat for hours, and I think we both benefit from it.

My younger two children had the same effect on me, although circumstances were different. I was so busy drugging and not doing the right thing that when I attempted to redirect my life, I had to be serious; making that type of lifestyle change required an ultimate commitment. Getting off drugs can be the difference between living and dying. So many people fall short through the process of completing the transition. When they don't hear from family, it can cause them to revert to the lifestyle. When they argue with family, it can cause them to revert also.

Relationship status (unfaithfulness or divorce) can also be a major contributor to a person failing to get clean. For me, the love of my children weighed heavy on my heart and mind. Their mother didn't bring them to see me for a long time, but I had to stay focused. I prayed hard because I knew as a father I had to represent

with my mind, my spiritual mind, and sometimes both. That was
if I really wanted to make an authentic difference in their lives.

Being very honest, in the beginning, I didn't know it as I
have written it here. That is the thing about having faith when it
comes to doing the right thing. I would actually feel pain in the
longing for my children, and when they came to visit me, I would
cry when they left. I had to have big picture thinking. A father's
love—a parent's love— runs deep. At least, it does for me.

Now I wonder how my father felt when Momma took us
away from him. How did that contribute to his alcoholism? Was he
even aware of the depth of his own pain? What happened? What
was he thinking as he saw us walking away from him on Irving
Street? The same with my stepfather Pete; what tragedy or impact
formed his level of understanding? How did he feel when Momma
broke up with him in 1979? It wasn't the first time…unfortunately,
for him it wasn't the last time either.

We are in the 21st Century and, as I previously stated, I've
been clean for quite some time. I had to endure my youngest
daughter turning her back on me for almost a year, because some
of life's core issues she has yet to experience. Initially, Sasha was
upset with me and I think I understand why, but I chose to avoid
any confrontation because I loved her. I wasn't very sure how to
address it, but that is behind us now. She is a lot like me, whether
she knows it or not, and she will prevail to her own level and type
of greatness.

Charles, Jr. is like me also; he has finally gotten a job and regardless, I love him, and I am proud of him because one day, just like with me, the light is going to turn on inside him, and he's going to know what it is that he is supposed to do.

Kychel has discovered her creativity, but she isn't sure which primary step will be the one she places her faith in. But, there is no doubt in my mind that when she does, she will be in the thick of it for real.

For now, all I can do is plant seeds. I have nothing tangible to leave any of them, at least not until I die. Not something pleasant to say, but it's the truth. Hopefully, with that being said, it will still be a long time before I give them anything significant…if you know what I mean.

Daddy was murdered in 1968. Seven years later, in 1975, my oldest brother, Paul Jr., was murdered. My sister, Leila, said that he was jumped. It seems that Junior started using heroin, had a habit and a bad enough tab. You can't owe in the drug game. The word on the street was that he used to take the drug dealers drugs from them. A year later, in 1976, my brother Tony, aka Kyleke, disappeared. Paul Jr. was battling his addiction and owed money to some local dealers. An overdose was forced on Junior. They gave him rat poison, waited for him to respond to the poison, and then started beating him up because they knew he could fight well. Functioning off a sober mind is one thing, but to try and maintain on drugs is an entirely different episode.

The legacy of men in the Smith family is horrible. To my understanding, my dad was an alcoholic. Junior was on heroin, I was on cocaine, and Tony stopped anything before it could be a habit, but I am not sure if the street life still led to his disappearance. *I had to change this; I've been clean from vices for almost twenty years now.* I need to let my children know that their lives don't have to consist of the things in this book. My son is a junior and I don't want the legacy for the Smith males, including my nephew, Aaron, to end up like the elder Smiths. I desperately want more for all my children. I want my son to pass on the family name and, more importantly, extend a positive legacy.

There were several occasions when I was really so scared. Pete tried scaring us into doing things. Maybe that's why I was a bed wetter, or maybe why I have such a vivid imagination, especially when it came to him telling us how he would teach us a lesson. He would try to make us believe that we should tell the family of any problems we had. As an adult I agree however, as a child, when we went to him we would still get into trouble with all the drama. I didn't agree with the way he handled situations. I would like to believe he meant well, and maybe he didn't know how to go about it. I have adapted many of his ways, and I am not happy of how I've turned however, there is a part of me that is very comfortable with who and how I am. I have some resentment from my childhood and that is why I had issues being around Pete at times. It's not an issue now, but it sure was a self-awareness process.

All of this father love talk leads me into realizing the fact that now that I am a father and grandfather, there are so many lessons to teach, and lessons to draw from for my own comfort in life. My father was actually murdered in '68; my oldest brother in '75; my closest brother disappeared in '76; I was heading out in '97/'98; it was an obvious pattern.

My God I am so grateful that I am still here and I can tell the story. I was setting my children up to be a number, a statistic in somebody's book that won't amount to anything. The responsibility would fall on my son. If the name was to be carried on with a sense of purpose, he would have to do it. My daughters may marry and none might be the wiser, but every man wants a son to lead a legacy. Most men want that even if they haven't taught their sons to do or be anything. I think it's a desirable feeling within a man to want his boy to have this sense of greatness about him.

Now it may very well be the daughters who make the difference (create or carry on the legacy), and I know that it's all-good. That's just not how we see things in our minds. All of my children are gifted. I don't know if they realize it, but on the strength that God put stuff, yeah that good stuff in me...I know some of it gets passed along, and I have no say on what it is...that is an actual gift to the world. As Enoch the 7th Prophet would

say, "Give thanks."

Chapter 8

EXPERIMENTING

I have always been highly sexual. My consciousness of sex, my desire for sex, being intrigued by women meant a lot to me. I have always wanted to be a furious lover. I can remember back to the sixties, when Motown was rolling. My older sisters, aunts and uncles got together and would have a good ole time. I distinctly remember the slow dancing—body to body—so close that you couldn't be any closer unless you were in each other's skin. The movement was so sensuous, and downright provocative.

I didn't know what the dances all meant, but I liked them, a lot. I would sneak a peek to see what they were doing. If we got caught looking, we were just told not to be so fresh or smart. That was the beginning of my interest and desire to explore my sexuality. I didn't just want to explore, but I wanted to know how it felt, how things worked.

I was in Brooklyn visiting with my family, and all of the kids were supposed to go play (as usual), because the adults were busy playing cards, drinking liquor, smoking cigarettes and doing things that I had not thought about discovering yet.

There were about seven kids. I was one of the only boys and one of the oldest amongst the others at the time. Well the oldest girl there (Mary) decided to play house. It wasn't my idea, but I didn't mind playing, especially since I was going to be the father. I figured I would not have to do much. Now I never played house before, and I really didn't know what I was supposed to do. I was into G.I. Joe, and straight up boy things. Therefore, I really didn't want to play with the other kids because they were younger than I was. At eleven years old, you feel like or wish you were a teenager.

Now I did have on this cool little outfit. You might remember that when you were young, your parents would always want to dress you up when you went out. Oh yeah, I also sported this cool little afro, that I was constantly reminded that if I wanted to keep it I had better not leave hair on the sink and I'd better take care of it. Meanwhile, back at the ranch, Mary was three years older than me, and she knew how to play house. The younger kids there were supposed to do what she said and I was supposed to be coming home from work. She would make believe that the kids were going to bed and she and I were going to bed in another room. I guess it is obvious to say that Mary must have liked me.

She kissed me and I got on top of her. Now I didn't know how this was supposed to work, but I didn't stop her; I let her lead. We both pulled our pants down and I wouldn't swear on a stack of Bibles, but that was my first time. Naturally, I began exploring with my own body, which I learned by listening to other kids and looking at my uncle's dirty magazines. My cousin and I would look at my uncle's *Screw* magazine anytime that he either left the house or was in the bathroom for a longtime. The next time that I actually had sex, I was fourteen or fifteen. I fed into the whole Scorpio thing; I had to be this and that when it came to sex and I sort of let that dictate my goals with girls. In many cases, it determined how I would act with them, how I felt about them, and what their role was with me. Peer pressure would help me define myself sexually.

I was a shy kid at heart, but I longed to be confident. I felt as if I was behind everybody else, especially when it came to social activities, recreational activities, academic activities, and style. I was a C student, I was introverted, and I had a high need of acceptance and no confidence at all. When other kids had PF Flyers, I had skips off the table on Third Avenue in the Bronx. When other kids wore Converse, I wore PF Flyers, and when they wore Pro Kids, I wore Converse. When it came to the girls, I was way behind the curve, and I didn't want to be behind nobody's curve.

Once I started high school, I started working part-time. I had this big Afro—no doubt; I could have been a Jackson. In fact, my best friend, Carlton, and I had the biggest Afros in our neighborhood. We were both Scorpios from DC, and both like the same musical groups. We would sing together just like the groups of our day. He could sing and played bass guitar. He was in a band called "The Liberators."

Carlton and I would listen to all the records and try to sing our favorites and talk about girls. During this time, I wasn't sexually active, but I am sure he was. I had a crush on a couple of his sisters, but it never really went anywhere. We went out with a pair of sisters from a church we were attending. I know he was getting some, but not me. I was kissing and that was about it. When I became a sophomore in high school, I began to catch up with the other guys. There wasn't a race, it was just puberty, I guess. Carlton and I did a lot of note comparisons on the young women during those years.

I remember when my sister, Monique, was about three or four years old, and I used to pick her up from the pre-k center. In many ways, education was a lot better back in the mid- to late 70s than it is now. In the Jackson's story, Joe Jackson told Jackie to fight a boy that was picking on him. The boy was jealous because Jackie and his brothers were growing very popular from the shows that they were doing. At that point in the Jackson's lives, they stopped spending time with their friends and started dedicating and devoting time to their craft. As a result, many other kids in the neighborhood felt slighted by the Jacksons. Joe jumped into the situation telling the bullies if they want to fight, they can, but to fight clean. He wanted his son to stand up and face his fears and not to be bullied around. Joe was a boxer and musician. Jackie was knocked down by the boy and his father told him don't be afraid, face that boy and kick his butt…and that is exactly what happened to me.

My girlfriend and I were being teased in the 'hood by a couple of guys (Clyde and Baby). As soon as my girl uttered one word to them, it was on. The two guys yelled out to me that they were going to get me. I told her not to say anything, but it was too late. I wasn't sure what to feel. I started practicing my martial arts more, I told my best friend. I didn't know what to do. I am not a fighter; I am a musician, a lover. That's who I am. However, the day would come when they would catch me alone.

It was a brisk fall afternoon and I was on my way to pick up my sister. Clyde and Baby had been getting high and drinking Old E (the best malt liquor/beer we had back in the day Old English 800). They saw me before I saw them. They told me straight up that they were going to beat me down, and they wanted my little sister to see it. I was scared to death, and nervous as hell. I had to figure out what to do, and fast. I had my hand in my pocket and I was holding on to my box cutter. I could have just started slicing, but that would delay me from picking up my four-year-old sister.

As soon as I got to the school, I called home. I spoke to Pete, and he came right away. I was thinking, *how in the hell do you get a yellow cab in Harlem, in no minutes flat? Especially when there are gypsy cabs all over the place.* He showed up in a cab, but I didn't see the guys. He told me that I had better tell him if I saw them, as the cab drove us back to Lionel Hampton, but before we actually got to the apartment, I saw both of those guys. Pete yelled, "Stop the cab!" We got out and it was on!

"Alright, who wants to fight my son?" Those were Pete's exact words. In fact, he did the same thing with my brother when he moved to New York from DC back in the 60s when my brother just didn't fit in and the locals wanted to bully him. Once I heard him yelling with so much exuberance, I was thinking, *When the hell did Don King show up? He was all loud with it, like we were selling tickets or something.* We didn't get into what happened we just got to the point. Clyde said, "I'll fight him," and we began dancing around, trying to feel each other out. He and I both threw a couple of punches. Baby said, "I'll fight him now." I was thinking, *Shit this ain't over now?* Baby was left-handed. He caught me with a couple of good shots to my face.

Pete yelled out, "He's left-handed and he's throwing bolos, can't you see them coming?" I am like no, I can't that's why they keep landing. I came back on Baby with a quick jab to his chest or maybe it was his jaw, but he said he didn't want to fight anymore. Clyde wanted another shot at me. I thought it was over, but Pete said, "Fight him Charles, let's get this over with." I immediately went into a martial arts stance. Bruce Lee had died a year or two prior and Clyde started making fun of me for being a Bruce Lee fan, and for switching up into martial arts instead of just street fighting. He started saying, "Bruce Lee is dead. Bruce Lee is dead." Clyde threw a punch, missed and I rushed him. I moved so fast that I didn't realize I had punched him in the eye. He said he

didn't want to fight anymore. Besides, we were fighting out in the

cold. When I went to school the next day and spoke to his

girlfriend, she said I had busted his eye.

·   I learned through that experience that sometimes you just

have to face a situation once and for all. Even when you are forced,

there can be a benefit to confronting your fears and challenges. I

also learned to have faith in my abilities, and I recognized that I

made good decisions (calling for help when unsure what to do). I

never had a problem from those guys anymore. I ran into them

again as an adult, but the past didn't seem to matter.

Fifteen years later, I was on Hamilton Terrace (about a

block or two from City College in Harlem), and I saw this guy

walking with a young lady, while pushing a baby carriage. I kept

staring at him because he looked familiar, and he seemed so

reluctant or unsure of me. It wasn't until five minutes later after

passing him that I realized it was Clyde. I also ran into Baby, but

you would have thought Baby and I were cut partners. We saw

each other, shook hands and hugged like it was all that.

I used to focus so much on being liked and fitting in. My

theory was that during these years I felt as if I was unimportant,

not popular, did not fit in, and my voice wasn't heard. Eventually, I

learned to accept not fitting in, because I would have a sphere of

influence. I also learned that I did not need a host of friends to have a meaningful life. The emotions that I experienced were natural; I just didn't understand them.

My sister, Cecelia, says that I can talk to the animals. I haven't tried talking to any animals, but if I did, I would want them to listen. If you were to ask me why I like talking and why I am so out spoken, I would tell you it is because of my childhood. I was the youngest. I didn't know what to expect from life, so I was quiet and tried to blend in. I was the follower, the meek one, the humble shy kid, but I always wanted to know why. Why this, why that, just why. My questions over the years were not answered to my satisfaction, in most cases. So, I am the animal that was created as a result.

My first experience of being dropped by a girl rocked my world. I never forgot it and I am finally learning from it. Without reason, a high school girlfriend didn't want to be bothered anymore. I never got a reason, and that bothered me quite a bit. I know that I wasn't very mature, and my feelings were fresh for the crushing. I didn't do anything silly, but I didn't know how to lead or how to fulfill my role in the relationship. I didn't know anything about how to have a girlfriend, so I lost the first one that meant something to me. I started going through the nice-guys-finish-last syndrome. The best part about that was that I made a commitment to myself that I would never be hurt again. I would guard my heart more cautiously for the rest of my life.

The next relationship was sort of a cushion. Truth is, after having my idealistic heart broken a few times, I decided I would prepare for future break ups by meeting someone else when things started going bad in a relationship, or setting my relationship up for failure so that I could be the victim. I played it safe anyway; I never went out of my way to get any girl. If she liked me and was attractive enough (meeting my criteria), she could be my girl. Effortless relationships are not good, because they don't equal happiness.

That's just a bit of advice for anyone interested in being happy in a relationship. You have to put effort into a relationship. If you are going to have to put effort into something, it might as well be something that generally interests you. If you want something special, you should go for it. Think about it. You are going to have to learn the person's likes and dislikes. When you want something or someone, you will enjoy what you want while you learn about it, because you are genuinely interested (in many cases not all…there are no guarantees).

For example, you meet someone and find out that he or she likes you more than you like him or her. You are not essentially motivated to be with the person, and spending "quality" time may be a secondary thought. You don't work hard to please them, because they're more vested than you. It is possible that things can change, but why gamble with your own personal happiness? It's easier to settle for what comes your way. Meanwhile, you are nice, maybe cordial, and you get used to being with that person. But there's no spark. There's a big difference.

At this point in my life, I was more turned on and tuned in to my natural desires (music). Carlton was hanging out with The Black Ivory, a very popular trio back in Harlem during the '70s. They made songs like "Don't Turn Around," "You and I," and "Mainline." Carlton was singing with the MLK Glee Club and he was enjoying some of the perks of being around the young celebrities. He told me about the exploits of the MLK Choir and all of the engagements they had. I wanted to be part of that life so bad. I left the group I sang with (Tears of Joy) and joined the MLK Fellowship Choir. Just joining the choir, I was very green with how things were done. I tried hard to fit in and wasn't sure of how to do it.

Carlton stopped coming to rehearsals, but I loved it. I was drawn like a bee to honey. I met a girl in the church that just had to have me escort her to her high school graduation and prom. This included breakfast and the whole nine yards. Her original escort couldn't take her for some reason or another, but I was the new kid on the block. In New Jersey they did it up. The graduation was held on the football field, the ball, which wasn't that impressive to me, was after, and they had a breakfast the next morning. It was really nice. Needless to say we started seeing each other. I had never been to a graduation held outside. Her friends were more diverse than I was at the time. I couldn't get into that pop-oriented culture, but the breakfast and all the private time was on point. I was graduating high school the very next year, so I knew what the whole experience was about.

We would sneak around to be alone, because as busy as we were, we never seemed to have time to be alone. In the beginning it was lots of fun as it always was. Her mom was an usher/missionary. Her father was a deacon, and her brother was in ministry also. I used to take a bus from the George Washington Bridge to see her (Route 4). I had to be careful of the schedule, so that I didn't miss my return trip.

Darlene and I did a lot of everything. I remember once we were at her home in Glen Rock, and I missed my bus home, all because of mischief. I lied to her dad, a deacon to get a ride home. Those were some crazy days.

Things started to fall apart between Darlene and me when she realized that she would be going to college away from home and our relationship could suffer some serious strain. She suddenly wanted us to see other people. I didn't agree, but that was what she wanted to do. I pulled back because I was hurt and I thought she was wrong. She felt she could have me anytime she wanted and other guys, too (not that it was all about sex, but at the time I didn't care what it was about, I just wasn't with that program).

The only reason I was in the choir was because of the way Carlton explained things to me. It seemed so exciting. He told me so many things about performing on the road and performing locally. I had a chance to get my feet wet with singing, and I learned so much. I learned about harmony, soloing, practicing, voice, rehearsals; it was just so much and I soaked it up like a sponge. I later found out that Darlene had previously gone out with one of my friends from the choir. He and I became close, but we butted heads from time to time. However, it didn't stop our male bonding; we remained cool way into our twenties or our thirties!

Another friend, Paul Laurence, who sung with the choir, was doing quite well for himself. Paul loved music and at a certain point, he stopped hanging out with us so much. He had been around long before I joined the group. Paul had aspirations of being a professional recording artist, producer, etc. He stopped getting high, and started reading up on the business. His group started doing a lot of shows during the '70s. He and I were cool, because of our alliance with music. He allowed me to go to some of his rehearsal and recording sessions. I supported many of his showcases around New York.

The group was a spin-off of his ensemble (LJE) at White Rock Baptist Church in Harlem. The group really had something to offer, and with Freddie Jackson on vocals, Paul and some of the others, it really made me feel special to be part of what was happening. Paul fit the '70s stereotype that we all fit—handsome with a nice Afro and he could sing, play the piano, and write music. I learned so much from him. I will never forget those early days.

The choir we sang with had several components. In addition to the choir, there was the ensemble, and a new splinter group called Soul Refreshment. At the time we were all young, very talented, and many of us were trying to find our way in life, deciding if we wanted to go to college, get jobs, be an artist, or do all of it. It was a rather complex time. I knew breaking up with a girl at that time was a lot for me to handle. I decided to protect my feelings and my heart, so I completely shut down. I didn't trust anyone too much at that time. My pain turned into anger, and that turned into determination.

Future relationships would flow with great desire, but also with much uncertainty. It would have been nice to know that *"When the student is ready, the teacher will appear."-anon.* Some relationships would be good, some would be bad, and some would be terrible. I didn't always realize why I did some of the things I did. I have met some nice girls in my life, but being afraid for my feelings was my worst enemy. After five to ten years of bad relationships or hurt feelings, the tone was set. I was probably my own worst enemy, but my feelings would remain guarded. I wanted so badly to love, but I really didn't know how. I was afraid to try to trust women and that was coupled with chronic drug use It just made my life a nightmare that I didn't even realize I was living. I went on to other relationships, not having very much success.

I think Odessa would be the next relationship that went awry. Pete once told me, "If you can count more than three friends on any hand that would be something special." I met Walter on my first day of college. Walter would eventually become one of my best friends. Walter was going out with a cutie named Stephanie and after he and I had gotten to know each other better, he introduced me to Stephanie's sister Odessa. She was the opposite of her sister. Stephanie was dark and lovely, Odessa was sort of a redbone version. She was a genuinely nice girl and I took total advantage of her. I was three and a half years older than Odessa, and I knew that she wasn't experienced. In fact, I was her new boyfriend at her sweet sixteen.

Eventually, after a relationship that didn't offer any growth, it was time for me to move on. Walter and I both had moved in with the girls and their mother (who had a heart of gold and a drinking PROBLEM to match). I wasn't mature enough to deal with Odessa the right way. I was still searching. After Walter and Stephanie had their problems, Walter moved out. Stephanie was preparing for college, and was hardly ever home. At first, it felt odd being there with Odessa and her mother, but then I had gotten used to it. Eventually I moved out, and Walter found out where I moved to and he and I became roommates.

Several flings later, I would run into my high school heartbreak donor. I came out of a breakup and into a rebound situation not showing any wisdom from my past. Drug use had been the culprit even when music wasn't an active part of my life. I probably should have been dating and not in a serious relationship during my late teens and maybe even early thirties. I have learned a lot about relationships and women during those experiences, but it wasn't until now that I can say that I really can benefit from what I learned about them.

As I look back over my life and think things over, I can truly say that I am blessed. I am a testimony. Just like the words of the song we have sung in church, true to life are those words. I wanted so desperately to be a lover boy when it was convenient, I wanted to have a girl that I felt I could relate to, and I wanted to be moving forward in the music business. The time wasn't right for me. I now know that I wasn't mentally prepared for everything that I wanted. I would repeat many of the same mistakes during my twenties and thirties. I have done a lot of soul searching in my life and it didn't amount to much of anything because I wasn't ready to grow.

Once again…*"When the student is ready the teacher will appear."* -anon

I have been a thinker all of my life, learning that when you are young, the only disadvantage to being a thinker is that you can't draw from any experience, because you have none. I did a lot of self-talk, only to find it wasn't time for me to have those answers.

"Self-talk can be good, but it's dependent upon what's happened, or what's happening. Self-talk can deteriorate one's perspective or destroy relationships. Don't assume you know because of the discussions that you have with yourself. Know because you have factored all necessary viewpoints (not just your own)."

—C. Cary

I know now that it was part of the learning process for my life, but after having a need of acceptance for so long, that changed and I started having a sense of entitlement. I went from one end of the spectrum to the other.

Trueality Enterprises

Chapter 9

GOOD / EVIL

Church life seemed so important to our family. I went to church every Sunday as a kid, even when I didn't want to go. As an adult, I go to church because I want to go and my life's philosophies have matured. As a teenager growing up in church and going through various experiences (some good and some not so good), we never knew when someone might call us to sing, pray or find a passage to start a service or anything like that. It would happen from time to time.

In addition to everything else, the music kept many of us off the streets during that time. My family has a strong background in the church. I surely wasn't going to change it. I know when I was younger I asked my mom why I had to go to church every Sunday. I told her it was the same message, at the same time of the year, every year. Her reply was more or less "Keep going; you'll find out why." So, I did. I attended a Mennonite church for many years. I didn't know it at the time, but it was the beginning of a multifaceted education, which I wouldn't realize until many, many years later.

As a Christian, you are supposed to love your neighbors as you love yourself. You are also supposed to forgive and forget. I must admit, I am still growing and learning. I got an early start with manipulating, getting over, hood life, and the works. Just think about it. When I was seven years old, I was roaming the streets for two weeks without anybody knowing what I was doing. I use to go to a neighborhood toy store and steal my favorite toys and all the accessories whenever I could. I stole money when it was convenient. As strange as it seems I didn't like to tell lies. I guess there was an inner battle going on with me as a *child* and Satan's recruitment crew. We did some stupid things. I can remember going to see *The Exorcist*, and after the film was over, two of my cousins (David and Bunny) and I were going to try to mug a woman with a fur coat.

I got a little nervous with that, so we dropped that idea. I don't know if it was demonic possession or what, but it was a weird night. I just happened to be carrying two toy guns that looked rather real. In those days, the level of detail was very good and there wasn't an orange or red tip in the muzzle of the gun. Our next target would be a yellow taxi. What a busy night that would be for a trio of eleven, thirteen, and fourteen-year-old kids from uptown. We got in a cab and told the driver of our destination, and after asking, "You know where we're going?" The driver starts to freak a little. He starts to complain about taking us and we eventually got out. Actually, he got so nervous it made me nervous. I kept saying, "Let's get another cab. Let's get another cab." Bunny was like, "No, shut up, let me handle this." I thought my gut instincts were kicking in to keep us from getting caught. *It was just a gut feeling, letting me know that it was wrong.* We were originally going to get a free ride, take the cab to our destination and hop out without paying.

Then, we tried another cab, and Bunny said, "We're going to rob the cab when we get out." We eventually get a middle-aged white man, wearing a golfer's cap. We tell him where we were going and he started to take us there. As we got closer to our destination, I was getting nervous. I knew that something was about to happen. Bunny asked for the guns to see which one looked more realistic. David was actually getting nervous (this was before the Diamond Dave we have all come to know and love was born to the street). We were about two blocks from the house. The driver was about to get robbed by three kids from the 'hood, and it was about to go down. Out of my nervousness, I tried to play everything off by saying, "I hope Aunt Esther got the money."

We pull up to the block. The driver said, "One of you wait here, while the others go get the money." I was so scared that I just ran. We all started running. The last thing I remember was the cabby yelling, "Freeze! Police!" I think that made us run faster. It was like the Mod Squad—two guys and a girl. We were uptown at the Dunbar Apartment houses, down the block from the Bill Robinson basketball court. There were exits and entrances all over the complex. I ran through the Dunbar, from 150th Street to 149th Street into the foyer of our grandmother's building. David ran right, but as he was making his exit, he saw Bunny fall down. She ran left and twisted her ankle.

He reluctantly went back for her. He had to; he couldn't leave his sister to get caught if there was a chance to help her. They hobbled through the Dunbar, scared and hurt. They made it to the foyer, and we were all glad, because if we left together we had to come back together. No exceptions. That was how it was in the old days. We went in the house and felt safe. We were all out of breath and nervous looking. Grandma Rose asked us what was wrong. In unison, we said "Nothing" with the quickness. We didn't get the money and we didn't get caught. It was a good day. Bunny's ankle had swollen considerably and she needed Epsom salt. There was none in the house. David was asked to go to the store. He didn't want to, so he asked me to go with him, and I said, "NO!"

The cops were probably out there looking for us. When we ran in, we heard sirens. I don't know what type, but we heard them. David and I were wearing the same exact Maxi style overcoats. Orange plaid, if you can believe that. He changed into his leather waist length jacket put on a cap. He went to the store ever so reluctantly. It made perfect sense to me. Why take a chance at being seen or getting caught? He made it back from the store without incident.

All other jobs from that point on would be a solo effort. We just wouldn't do any criminal activity together. Regardless of how scared we all were, the three of us had experience as the victim and as the assailant. We all knew another thing, that if our parents or grandparents had any idea, we would definitely catch hell. If Tony found out, it would have been all over for us. He was the closest one to all sides of the family, especially when it came to trouble.

The family would have probably asked my brother why he didn't stop us, or what he knew about it. I felt good about the little shit I did. I thought that it was okay as long as I didn't hurt anybody or anything. What it did do was build up a false confidence within me about my sinful or wrongful ways. I would take certain chances because I had never been caught. I figured you couldn't prove what you don't know. I was old enough to know the things I did were wrong, but I did them anyway. There was no excuse. There were so many situations that I can recall, as far back as grade school when we thought stealing bubble gum from the newspaper/shoeshine stand was being slick. We all knew better.

If I thought I would get caught I didn't do it. I had the mindset that if you didn't get caught that meant you were good at what you were doing. I learned that was true and false. It seems that all of the things that I had gotten away with came back to haunt me later or harder in my life. What goes around does come back in one way or another. You would have to do a tremendous amount of good to offset the bad and even then, you are still accountable for your actions.

—C Cary.

Trueality Enterprises

Eventually I discovered the Baptist church. WOW! I was shocked with all that rhythm, emotion and inspiration. I never wanted to go to any other type of church. The Mennonite music wasn't bad, but after spending so long in the Mennonite churches this was refreshing. At fourteen years old we moved. I didn't want to move, but when I did, an entirely different life was opened up to me. Puberty, independence, spirituality, religion and God's gifts and talents were just a few of the revelations that I learned about. It was the beginning of my education.

Life 101 is what I would call it if it were a class. I started going to Baptist churches regularly. Other than the people, I didn't particularly miss going to the Mennonite churches anymore. I met some friends in my new neighborhood. They not only went to Baptist churches, but they also sang in the choirs. I was in awe. Thank goodness I became close friends with them. I loved the Jenkins family as if they were my own family. I wanted to spend all of my time with them. I had a crush on the oldest sister, then I started liking the sister that was my age and I even felt the younger sister, Cynthia, was a looker.

It's sort of difficult to explain, but I also looked at the girls as friends with no strings attached. They each were so talented. I imagine they are still talented. Had it not been for them, I may have never had the opportunity to sing in church. The first time I sang a solo in church, I was with the Jenkins family, and the first group I joined was at Ebenezer Baptist on 8th Avenue off 132nd

Street with the Jenkins family and they encouraged me to pour it all in.

The oldest boy (Carlton) and I had a lot in common. I joined the group that he sang with also and at that point in my life, I really started to learn about girls and the game of boyfriend and girlfriend. It would happen eventually, but I am glad I learned in an environment that also helped me to grow as a young man. I was in church so much I guess it only made sense that I started looking for a church home. I found out so much about churches, congregations, pastors and musicians. It blew my mind when I found out about the gay society in church. It blew my mind even further when I found out a lot of the people in our group were gay. I knew about gay people, but I had no exposure to the gay lifestyle and if would affect me. I was cautious.

I started working part-time, once I got into high school. I had this big Afro—no doubt I could have been a Jackson. In fact, Carlton and I had the biggest Afros in our neighborhood. We were both Scorpios, we were both from DC, and we both liked the same music groups. We sung together, just like the groups of our day. He sang and played bass guitar. He was in a band called "The Liberators."

Carlton and I would listen to all the records and try to sing our favorites and talk about girls. During this time, I wasn't sexually active, but I'm sure he was. I had a crush on a couple of his sisters, but it never really went anywhere. We went out with a pair of sisters from a church we were attending. I knew he was getting some, but not me. I was kissing and that's about it. When I became a sophomore in high school, I began to catch up with the other guys. There wasn't a race, it was just puberty. Carlton and I did a lot of note comparisons on the young women during those years.

I would sing all of the parts to any song I liked. It could have been soprano parts, bass parts, soloist or groups. If I liked the song, I'd learn it and sing it. I just knew better than to interrupt George (pianist and music director). I sang while at the Mennonite church, but let's say it didn't start with purpose until I started singing in Baptist churches. The Tears of Joy consisted of Kathy, Kevin, John, Cynthia, Shelley, Carlton, Roland (keyboard player/director) and me. Their brother Billy attended, but he didn't sing with us. The church was First Ebenezer Baptist Church. We had quite a few engagements. That was really good for me. I was still pretty shy at that time. During rehearsals, we'd go over a song and somehow I started singing the solo part. They all convinced me that I sounded nice singing the song. My first solo was André Crouch's "Take Me Back."

The Jenkins family was definitely talented. The siblings were mostly musical, but also athletic. We would have jam sessions in the back room of their house. Carlton played bass guitar and sang, Cynthia played flute, danced and sang, Shelly sang and danced, Kevin played drums and sung background, and I sang with them from time to time. During this time, I was beginning to know the family well. Carlton became my lifelong best friend.

First I joined the Martin Luther King Fellowship Choir, and then I joined the Martin Luther King, Jr. Ensemble Movement. It was odd how things played out because Carlton was telling me about these different experiences, and how much fun it was. So you could say I joined the group because of him, and Carlton became less involved until he eventually left the group. He continued to sing in the Martin Luther King Glee Club.

The Fellowship Choir and the ensemble sang all over the place—every local or major church in New York, New Jersey, Connecticut, and Pennsylvania. We sang at Lincoln Center, The NYC Port Authority and at cotillions in the New York area. After joining the MLK Ensemble, there were opportunities to expand musically. That opportunity finally came because founding members—Gene, his sister Tracy, and Valerie—left to pursue other options. The group sang at various churches in Harlem on Saturdays. There would be tourists from all over the world visiting New York, and they would visit some of Harlem's oldest churches.

I learned so much about music, as well as stage presence. The MLK Ensemble recorded an album prior to my arrival in the group. We sold copies of the album and got a percentage after so many performances. It was one of the best early musical experiences for me. I'd occasionally get a solo of "Oh Happy Day" or "He Calmed The Ocean." At times, there would be busloads of people early Saturday afternoon waiting to be entertained. I've been fortunate to have people really care about me. As I sit here and think about it, a broad smile covers my face.

Carlton's brother Billy and I went to a Caribbean dance uptown near JFK High School and we had a good time. After the dance was over, we took our girls to the bus stop, and then proceeded to the train station. We walked by a bar casually en route to the train and about three or four big white guys came out. This was one of the first times that I encountered a fearful situation; I was about fourteen years old. The men that taunted us were in their early twenties. I didn't know if it was a racial thing, an intimidation thing, I just couldn't explain the attack.

As we passed the bar, we were talking about the girls. Now picture this, it's during the seventies, we were wearing big-collared colorful shirts with the collar on the outside of the jacket, knit or gabardine slacks, I was sporting a big Afro and probably, platform shoes. One of the men yelled out something to us as we ditty-bopped to the station. My friend yelled back to the guy, "I don't know what you're talking about. I'm looking good." We laughed.

I decided to look back and saw them running behind us. I yelled to Billy, "Let's go!" We took off. Man, you are talking about scared? We got no more than two blocks away, and Billy said, "I'm not running no more." I was shocked; my thinking is man you better come on. I ain't letting anybody catch me to jack me up, especially a posse! Billy was ready to take a stand. I continued to run around the cars and they told me that if I didn't stop running they were going to hurt Billy. I felt horrible, but I wasn't ready to get caught. They had Billy up against a building, pushing and punching on him. I was so scared that I really didn't know what they were doing to him. I eventually stopped. One of the guys pushed me up against a car. He clinched his fist and drew it back to let me have it.

When he hit me I thought he had a pillow in his hand. I guess they wanted to scare us, because it seemed as if they were throwing haymakers, but there was no power.

I fell to the ground and one of the guys kicked me. I was doing quite a bit of acting, but they really didn't hurt us. I couldn't figure what was the point. Bill told me later that one of the guys told him that he didn't want to do this, but he had to because of his friends.

When I stood, the guy held me up against the car. I was scared, but started to realize maybe it wasn't as serious as I initially thought. Nearby, there was a black man going into his trunk. I believe he saw the whole thing. He yelled out, "Hey! Leave those kids alone." They responded, "Mind your business." He yelled out again. The men left us alone and went over to him. We had a chance to get away.

We started to run away, but just before we left the area, Billy looked to see what was going on with the man who verbally defended us. Billy said, "They're beating him up, Charlie." Now I had to be scared, because I didn't even want to look back, I wanted to take advantage of every second to get away. When it came to Billy and I, there was a strong possibility that the men were trying to put fear in us, but with the man that spoke up for us, I think he may not have been so lucky. We went to Billy's uncle and told him what had happened. His uncle lived a block away. Uncle Charlie grabbed his aluminum baseball bat and walked us to the train station. There was no sign of our rescuer. Uncle Charlie had no fear; he had his bat, he was in his neighborhood, and I imagine he could handle himself. That was the first time I was literally afraid for my life.

We didn't see the black guy who tried to help us; only the white guys who tried to beat us down. The next day we were able to look back on this situation rather lightly, but that evening was no joke.

I learned and continue to learn that life is a process of continuous learning. With fear, it can be so extremely hard to know that your decisions at that time are right. The reason for that is because of your feelings and emotions. When you have adrenaline pumping much faster than it does on a regular basis and all of your senses are on overdrive, it can be challenging to make a sound decision, unless you are   used to make decisions under pressure. Ninety percent of your life is lived in your head. By that, I mean our thoughts determine our actions, but not only do our thoughts determine our actions they also determine our fears, insecurities, uncertainties, and assumptions. We sometimes will go through an entire episode in our heads not having much solid evidence of why we think and feel that way. Imagine liking or not liking someone (friend or family) totally based on assumption.

That is so powerful, but can you use it to the best of your abilities. Just think about it when you are alone. Knowing you have the ability to change that mind set and you can be in a position to make better decisions. Sometimes we have to learn, and learn to get used to thinking outside of ourselves and by that I mean it was a good idea to consider the actions and sometimes the feeling of a hand full of people versus an entire race, nation or culture.

Every Christian, Jew, Moslem/Muslim, Buddhist or Hindu does not share the same viewpoint. Their views may be the same regarding their culture, religion, or general beliefs (generally speaking), but even then there can be differences in how some things are approached. That is why it isn't good to judge a mass of people by the actions of a few. We are still all different regardless to what beliefs we may share. Other areas notoriously known to be fearful are public speaking, singing, addressing an audience and fitting in. However, if you are the person confronted with this issue, your opinion may vary.

I didn't tell my parents everything about that night, probably, because I didn't want them to try and stop me from hanging out with the Jenkins clan. I was too embarrassed to say, "We got beat up last night." I did learn a valuable lesson about fear, race, and choices.

It's ignorant to decide the value of an entire race based on the actions of a few. Just because those guys chased us down and tried to beat us up, or scare us, doesn't mean that all white people should be judged or that all white people don't like black people. I feel that is an irresponsible decision and mindset to hold on to. I have known many white people in my time that have not treated me that way.

Regarding fear and choices… although I was afraid, I understand that in some cases you may have to take a stand. Sooner or later, you must address your fear no matter how great it is. The lesson in that is that you may find your fear is something that can be overcome.

Chapter 10

BUGGING OUT

Even back in the day fitting in was related to several things. Going anywhere popular that was a way of fitting in. Celebrity sightings were another way of fitting in or being down. Having the latest hairstyles or clothing was definitely a way of fitting in. I wasn't in any of these categories for a long time. Plus when you add in the fact that I wasn't a native New Yorker and I had to learn the way of the streets. That was a lot of pressure for a kid from Chocolate City. The family moved from 147th Street and 7th Avenue to 130th Street and St. Nicholas Avenue. We moved into a new development called The Lionel Hampton Houses. It was 1974 and the girls were starting to take an interest in me and I was taking an interest in them.

I seem to have eyes in the back of my head at this point because every girl that I thought was interesting or attractive…I saw them. It wouldn't matter if they were too old for me, or just right. Now if I could just learn how to get my parents to loosen the reigns so I could hang out like the rest of the blossoming teenagers. I was still new to the neighborhood and just started going out with Renay. These two guys from the block were talking smack as I walked to the bus stop, and Renay turned around and asked with attitude, "What y'all looking at?" They knew who I was because of the friends I'd recently met.

Having it all together isn't necessarily all that it's cut out to be. You

can look sharp, smell good, and have that twinkle in your eye, but you are

prone to have problems, just like anybody else.

Think about the lyrics to the song that Barbara Streisand sings, "People,

who need people are the luckiest people in the world." Babies need their

parents, students need their teachers...even Hercules needed Zeus.

—-C. Cary

They promised to kick my ass. I knew not to say anything, because the timing was wrong. They scoped me out over the next couple of days. I stayed in the house trying to get my head together. I wasn't sure what the proper approach would be, but I knew I had to fight. I always loved and greatly respected Martial Arts. I kept a handbook with moves and techniques close by, hoping to not need them. My mentors were Muhammad Ali, Bruce Lee, Jim Kelly, Chuck Norris and Ron van Clief. Now I wasn't a fighter, but the pugilist that I respect most, were the people that I could identify with.

I was never an out and out bad kid, but I guess I experimented with negative behavior from time to time. By the next year I would be given permission to smoke reefer in my room as long as the smell wasn't all over the house. I would burn incense or spray air freshener. My stepfather was the second or third person that I would smoke reefer with. Mom didn't like it one bit. She would tell me time and time again, "You don't need to be smoking that stuff". She'd say things like, "Your body is a temple, a temple that God gave you, and you have to take care of it". I knew that she was right it just felt good doing something different. I enjoyed the sensation and the mechanics of getting high. It's simple yet interesting. I was cleaning the weed, breaking down the buds if any, fixing the paper and rolling it up. I'd come a long way from hating the smell.

Whatever doesn't kill you makes you stronger.
—*anon*

I dare do anything wrong or improper, I had to remember, **Pete will bust my ass wide open.** Heck of a thing for a kid to remember. This was especially true if you are the type of kid that has a vivid imagination. I guess it's something you can get over, or do you? I don't know, maybe that's why I am twisted right now. If I didn't get a beating I was put on punishment. That was supposed to be a real payment for my wrong doings. I imagine mom tried to do what she thought was best at the time, as far as supporting her husband and his disciplinary strategies.

As an adult my cousins would remind me, Charlie you always got a beating or you always seemed to be getting in trouble. I don't know if I blocked it out, but I do remember a lot of not so good times growing up. I do know that I didn't want to do to my kids some of the things that were done to me.

It was around February 1979 and my cousin Renee was staying with us for a while and there seemed to be a lot of tension in the air, more often than not. I picked up reefer for Pete and we'd smoke together. I was buying my own too. Anyway, one day while all seems well, Mom, Renee (my cousin), Monique and I are all home. Pete starts talking loud and talking about the past. He was crying, and I assume feeling angry. Suddenly, he starts rambling off about his mother and grandmother. I think he was banging on the bedroom doors trying to get someone to listen, then later he tried to provoke everyone. He called Renee all types of names and made accusations about her. He opened my door, got in my face and tried to make me take a punch. It was a loud and confusing situation.

The whole time this was happening he was smoking reefer and drinking wine. He actually flipped before our eyes and ever since then he seemed to feel real comfortable being seen that way. I never totally bought it, but he played the cards…if you know what I mean. He finished his wine and started melting different colored crayons over the bottle. You had to see it…crazy on one hand and very artistic on the other. We all remained very quiet for a while. My mother whispered to me not to say a word to him. I was scared and angry. I just didn't know what to do. The guys on his job even notice how he changed. They started calling him crazy Pete. One day he had an accident at work. Why did he have to get hit on his head? He was already bugging. In another incident, he cursed out a colleague and a supervisor. People at his job started calling him crazy Pete, and as a result, he was forced into retirement. My mom insisted that nothing confrontational should happen between Pete and me. I swear there was a few times I just wanted to snuff him real bad.

Chapter 11

BEYOND COLLEGE

Pete needed an excuse to lash out and he wanted me to be it. I'd started college at this time and was trying to get together. Once this happened I knew I wouldn't be able to get my head into the books under that type of pressure. Walter, Craig and I were all having problems with our parents at that time. They received grants or loans to go to school. All I got was money for books. After two semesters, things just fell apart. My mom asked me about moving out to get away from Pete and his sporadic, violent tendencies. I spoke to a couple of guys about what I was going through. Walter and I made a decision to move. I told my mother what my plan was, so that she would be comfortable and not worry. She took my sister Monique and moved to Washington with my other sister Cecelia. I moved to the Bronx with my friend Walter.

On the first day of college I was on the train and I saw this guy looking at me. He had a reddish tint Afro and he had sort of a nervous smile on his face. We kept making eye contact. I guess we were both a little nervous and unsure of where we were going. When we got to our train stop, we both stood up to get off. Now, I wasn't sure if he was one of those guys that started trouble, because I stared at him or what but we both left the train and went separate our ways. I finally found my first class on campus, I had no idea how big the campus was, and had no idea I would once again run into the guy from the train. His name was Walter.

Walter was from the Bronx. We became good friends. I was also in college with friends from junior high, high school and church. Once again, as I look things over I feel that there were too many past associations in my present.

During my college transition, I lived at home still. It was hard to get it together when it seemed like all Pete needed was an excuse to lash out at me. Once this happened, I knew I wouldn't be able to get my head into the books under that type of pressure. Walter, another friend Craig and I were all having problems with our parents at that time. They received grants or loans to go to school. All I got was money for books. My mom asked me about moving out to get away from Pete and his sporadic, violent tendencies. I spoke to a couple of guys about what I was going through. Walter and I made a decision to move. I told my mother what my plan was, so that she would be comfortable and not worry. She took my sister Monique and moved to Washington with my other sister Cecelia while I worked on a way to bring my plan to fruition.

Many of us were not having a good transition. We collectively messed up. We played cards, got high, messed around with the girls in school, and drank. After about two semesters we all got together and decided that we'd leave school. I didn't get much financial assistance from the government, because I told my family to be honest on the applications. Most if not all of my friends were getting money for their classes and for their books. Had I known how it worked, I would have lied on my application just like everybody else. I got nothing. I felt you should be honest, so I took the fair route and became the square.

We all left under a leave of absence or something that we hoped would keep the door open. Some of my friends got jobs. Walter and I got an apartment in the Bronx. He and I were pretty tight. Walter, Craig, and a bunch of us left school around the same time. Everyone was having problems adjusting to the notion of being a professional student on track to graduate college and deal with the real world. For some of us it was our mom, or our dad, or not having money, but everyone was being tested. The truth of the matter was I wasn't ready for college and with Pete bugging at home. I simply couldn't focus. I would rather play cards in the lounge, or get high in between classes, and I wouldn't make the cut.

At that time I initially remained very active with the choir and the ensemble. Now Walter and I were really good friends, but Lord knows we've had our differences. We lived up on Tiebout Avenue and 183rd Street. He had received a settlement from a car accident that had occurred years prior to our meeting, but it couldn't have happened at a better time. He looked out for his homeboy. Since we had just left college, I moved out and needed an income. We actually went to a job agency, and he bought two jobs; one for each of us. Walter's family lived around the corner and with us. I got to know who everybody was and where everything was in the neighborhood.

Tony, Carl, Skip, Darryl, Wayne, Jamel…it's been awhile since I've seen some of the brothers, but they're still the brothers. It was very uncomfortable for me in the beginning. I had to learn multiple personalities and this is where I'd lay my head, so it was home. I was adopted as a brother into the Hayes family. The boys were cool, just a little on the wild side. Carl sold loose joints every morning before school; Darryl was trying to follow behind Carl. Wayne was the baby, who wound up making babies. He looks just like Walter. Terrell would kid around a lot. Walters' father took me in as a son, and the streets would eventually take him away a few years later. It seemed like everywhere I went, every effort I made; God was watching and protecting me during my twenties.

We didn't have that place for long. I was a rookie bachelor fresh out of the nest trying to be a man. When I lived in the Bronx in those early days I knew what time it was, but I just wasn't refined. I smoked so much Angel Dust one night it was just crazy. I went back and forth from Manhattan to the Bronx. It was around three o'clock in the morning and the music was blasting. I was amazed to find myself sitting on my bed crying, asking an ambiguous question over and over again, "Where's my brother"? Dust can do that to you. It wasn't my first dust trip and it wouldn't be my last.

Walter worked downtown and he moved out. My Mother had previously separated from my stepfather and moved to Washington but at this time she was considering moving back to New York with my sister. She came to visit me and began to make her plans to move back to the big city. I was looking at another place not too far from the Yankee Stadium.

During this time I was embarking on a new career. I worked with the city of New York for about a year as a verification clerk with Housing Preservation & Development. That year was a learning experience as a young black man in corporate America. Before I landed the position, I had to be tested. I took all the tests that were needed. I didn't know what the difference was between a civil service position and a provisional position. The woman in charge of hiring and training was a strong black woman by the name of Ms. Emma Mustgrave. She was very hard on me. I thought my youth and good looks would carry me, but it didn't. I dressed casually, not professionally for work. I didn't bring a pen or a notebook to take notes.

There were at least a dozen provisional employees and I was the only unprepared person there. It was really rough for me in the beginning. Ms. Mustgrave spoke to me very harshly and gave me lots of attitude. I actually started to quit. I started thinking really hard about what was going on. Why was this woman speaking to me so harshly, and why did she seem to have such disdain for me? What was it about me? I am young, I am handsome; everybody else seems to like me. Right? Wrong! I realized that I was 19 years old and adulthood was knocking on my front door. I wasn't living with my parents and this was truly the beginning of living life on life's terms.

I decided to speak to Ms. Mustgrave privately. I asked her if I could see her, and she said yes. I told her that I realized why she was so tough on me. I let her know that I respected what she was doing, because I realized that I had to grow. She smiled and from that point on everything was literally ok. She smiled because I got it, I don't think she figured that I would catch on, but I did. I stayed there for about a year or so and people all around me were getting laid off. I seemed to be untouchable. I'll attribute that to God working through Ms. Mustgrave.

God gives us opportunities, but he also sends messages for us to take advantage of. I realized after a few days that Ms. Emma didn't have anything against me. Ms. Mustgrave wanted me to be a responsible person; she also wanted me to be ready for Corporate America). I was very proud of my progress and I know today that I only had God to thank for it.

I left my city job and started working in the banking industry as a teller. I would eventually go from being a bonded commercial banker to a savings banker. Mom moved back to New York and resumed her career with Nynex, and Monique started school.

I began meeting many people of different backgrounds, and I even met the mother of my first child. Actually, I had my sights set on a few women, but when I saw her I just had to get to know her. She was from Brooklyn and I thought she was fine as hell.

I knew Brooklyn girls, but the only one I was ever interested in was a high school crush, this was different. I had to get to know her and I felt I was ready for someone different. I remember when Kim first started working at the bank. She had great energy, and she was very friendly. She came across as really down to earth. She was model tall, dressed very nicely, and I just had to get her attention. Finally, I did and it would be a slow process to the goal. I actually had to date her, and I wasn't ready for that, but that's how it was. After a few weeks maybe a month, I got her to come by my apartment, but she wouldn't have sex with me. We took slow walks to my apartment; we'd stop at the deli and get fresh deli sandwiches and a couple of Lowenbrau's.

After a few more weeks, it happened totally unexpected. I was shocked, but we began to see each other exclusively. As we began to learn each other I found that she was so outspoken that we couldn't get along. There were so many times that we'd argue, make up, and repeat the cycle over and over again. I wasn't ready for a child, but when the seed is planted, it shall grow, my first child Kychel was born. I wouldn't or couldn't realize that I wasn't mature enough to except the responsibility of fatherhood. I was getting high all the time; I was gigging with my band, and too immature to compromise. Kim actually thought that I was messing around, but as God is my witness...I wasn't messing around. I'd hang with the fellas, and that was it. Kim and I argued many days, and nights. We'd argue violently too. We lived together in the Bronx 751 Gerard Avenue, on the 3rd floor, one block from Yankee Stadium.

After being falsely accused, and having over a dozen arguments about it, an opportunity presented itself one day and I foolishly took advantage of it. I moved out. I left Kim at home with my mother and my newborn daughter. I couldn't deal with the fighting anymore. I was glad to walk away, but I actually felt my daughter's need for me so many times. It hurt so deeply that I wouldn't go visit her like I was supposed to because every time I left it hurt deep.

I was so into my band, and I loved every minute of it. I also used my music to bury the pain. Saturday's and Sunday's we'd rehearse from two o'clock until eight o'clock faithfully. I had an affair with my female lead vocalist that lasted a couple of years and of course there was another break up. I thought my female vocalist would be my wife. We made love all the time, we played music, and got high. She could dance, she was cute, and she had a pretty nice vocal range, but that wasn't enough and it wouldn't last.

As a result of my past relationships, I understand why people hurt each other the way that they do. I am not saying that I condone ignorance in relationships, but I truly feel that I understand why we treat each other so cruel. I know men that have actually been turned off from women because of the various differences (Mars and Venus). I am not gay and I thank God for not being gay, because everything doesn't have to be experienced in order for us to know what is and what isn't for us. I'd like to feel that I am sympathetic and empathetic without having had to walk that route.

At that time I lost touch with Walter, I later found out that he moved to DC.

Just like a person can feel that they are/were driven to hurt, steal, lie, take or cheat because someone cornered them with words, pressure, actions, or whatever, the reality is you don't ever have a real reason to do wrong, but we are all human and sometimes our weakness gets the best of us. Those are the times when we really need to think before we act (to thine own self be true). Anger and frustration seem to be the most common emotions that people use when it comes to placing fault on others. It seems that it was necessary for me to go through those hard times. The many experiences that I've encountered, I've been able to learn from them. I realized that it helped me have the outlook I have today. I can make healthy choices today whereas in the past I would repeat many of the same mistakes over and over again.

Frustration

Frustration isn't anything more than a reaction. The situation doesn't cause frustration. Rather, you choose to be frustrated by it. And as such, you can choose to transcend your frustration. Realize there is always something you can do, even if that something is just to accept the situation as it is.

Frustration is useful because it helps you identify things that need changing and improving. It helps you understand what you want, what you don't want, what works, and what doesn't.

Welcome your frustrations for what they can teach you. Then move on past them, and take the actions that they indicate. Once you are aware of the problem, frustration is of no use. Discard your frustration, knowing that you are in control.

You know it's really odd how we learn. All living things, act, react or respond. We (humans) are not very different. Like changes in life, we usually don't embrace change. Like learning in life, we prefer to learn from positive experiences and shy away from the negative. True learning comes from both positive and negative.

"Learn to embrace change" –C. Cary

Chapter 12

REAL LIFE

I struggled from time to time trying to act normal, but the disappearance of my brother really bothered me. Meanwhile, I stayed active in school, church and in the neighborhood. I waded through life, and various experiences with getting high and partying even in my brother's absence. Time waits for no one. I felt, wow I am getting older. I have my music, and I have my freedom. I started dating a girl from the group MLK. She was a nice girl from New Jersey with these really pretty eyes, and a pair of the deepest dimples you would want to see. She had her mind made up that she liked me. Initially I didn't know. She was graduating from high school and her date couldn't make the graduation ceremonies.

In New Jersey they did it up. They had the graduation, the ball was after and they had a breakfast the next morning. It was really nice. Needless to say we began seeing each other. The graduation was held outside on the football field, and it was pretty nice. I had never been to a graduation held outside. The ball wasn't that impressive to me. Her friends were more diverse than I was at the time. I couldn't get into that pop oriented culture, but the breakfast and all of the private time was on point. We would sneak around to be alone, because as busy as we were, we never seemed to have time to be alone. In the beginning it was lots of fun as it always is. Her mom was an usher, and or missionary. Her father was a deacon, and her brother was in ministry also. I use to take a bus from the GW Bridge, to see her (route 4). I had to be careful of the schedule, so that I didn't miss my return trip.

As a teenager I played the field off and on it. I remember seeing at least 3 girls at the same time. What a scoundrel I was. I juggled two girls from Jersey and one from Little Rock, Arkansas. One of my Jersey girls would pick me up and take me out to New Jersey, or to the beach. The Little Rock girl was nice, but she was just something to do, and of course my main girl, I saw her pretty regular too. Did I say what a scoundrel? It didn't happen often, but I had my moments.

I couldn't stand being in the middle of some mess, but I guess what comes around goes around in one way or another. I learned later that my girl used to go out with someone else from the group (Gene). He was mad cool when we hung out, but he was the alpha male and I was the new kid on the block. The first time I tried blotter he and I were together. In fact, when the crack epidemic hit, Gene and I were as thick as thieves.

We had a seriously tight crew. We were all trying to find ourselves. It was Gene, Tanya, Tracy, Darlene, Pip, Valerie, and I. Evaluating the crew, I would say we were the borderline crew. We were the ones that didn't stay in church from sun up till sun down. We had to learn how to cut those corners for our frequent mischief. Looking back even deeper, maybe there was some other reason why this crew was formed. We loved to party, and we did plenty of it. We were all in high school almost all of us in church and all down. We'd go to Gene and Tracy's house because they had cable with all the stations, and besides that, we were homies. We had endless good times as teenagers. We'd go to concerts to see Earth, Wind & Fire at Madison Square Garden or Cameo at Radio City.

Over the years Gene and I hung out no matter what. On another note I either worked full time in the summer or I worked in the summer youth program. I had to have money. *My drug use wasn't to be taken lightly* even though I was only EXPERIMENTING. I guess this is what happens when we exercise our freedom of choice. This was the beginning of a very long and enduring lesson. There is no coincidence or is there?

After losing a college bound girlfriend, it was hard for me to fully commit to a relationship. I learned my lesson early in life that the opposite sex isn't to be trusted, because the opposite sex will screw you (feelings and all). *Of course this isn't true for everybody, or all the time, but unfortunately it seems to happen naturally to many of us enough of the time.* It also has to do with the loneliness I experienced as a child, and how I dealt with it. I was aware when my brother would run away from home, when my mom left us to set up a new life in New York.

I know life isn't about vengeance, but I sure feel better when someone who did me wrong would have the tables turned on them. It was 1978 and all was great. I continued being Mr. Celebrity in school, singing in church and hanging with my boy

Carlton because of our similar interest. Years later I would try to get Carlton to sing in a group with me, and Gene. We rehearsed a few times in between my get high sessions with Gene, but it wouldn't work.

I was fairly popular in school because of my singing, but I didn't have a date for the prom. I decide to ask a girl that I liked, but it was said that she got around, and I didn't know if it was true or not. I asked her and she said yes. The girl I really wanted to take I couldn't. She was from Brooklyn too and had a very possessive boyfriend to match her beauty. I was forward yet still really shy in so many ways. I guess you could say that I was an opportunist with the opposite sex. If I was attracted to a girl I might let her know, but if she came on to me that would be fine too. I was afraid of the rejection.

Once we were sure we were going to graduate some of the guys hung out and all night. Billy Taylor, Eddie Byrd, George Andino, and there was somebody else from the Bronx along with myself. We got fired up. We had Panamanian Red, Acapulco Gold, Colombian, Chunky Black, Cocaine and Dust. Eddie got sick and we took him home. The rest of us stayed out and came to school in a yellow Marathon taxi. One of the cab drivers from that night before was a man by the name of Calvin Nesbitt. Billy & I would run into Mr. Nesbitt from time to time. He would let us smoke refer in his car, but he always tried to instill some wisdom.

Our graduation was held at Carnegie Hall. My mom and Pete showed up with Aunt Lorraine (Sweet Lorraine). She always called me Sweet Charlie. I took pictures with everybody that I could, especially those that I knew. I was still feeling very lonely on the inside. I was asked to sing with Norman Thomas High School choir. Ramon Reeburg was the director of the choir and was pretty well versed musically. I knew him from the outside church circuit as well as the school music teacher. He asked me to sing because the male section was lacking a little.

After the graduation ceremonies I double dated with a buddy that I really wasn't close to; we took a couple of girls to Jack's Nest on 23rd Street. It wasn't fun. It was also an indication of how fleeting sentimental moments can be. After four years of closeness, searching ourselves, and preparing to walk out into the world and take it on…it went flat. One hour after graduation for me, it went flat.

For Prom night I rented a tuxedo and a limousine. I picked up my date that lived in Brooklyn hoping she would be impressed by this grand gesture. I liked her, but really didn't want to take her out because, although I had a part time job... I didn't have a lot of money. Our prom was at the Waldorf Astoria. We had another impromptu prom at a club called Pippins. I planned to start college in the fall of 1978.

Chapter 13

GETTING HIGH

As a teen I started buying marijuana. I bought it for Pete, as well as myself. I even sold it in high school for a short period of time. I was reckless in those days. I rolled a joint in my favorite English teacher's class and almost got caught. My hang-out partner, Geoff, and I were on a mission when we hung out. We had a lot of good laughs. We would go to clubs like The Garage or The Buttermilk Bottom and party for hours. We dug those Mike Stone parties. Acid anyone? I would go out to Brooklyn meet Geoff; we'd play music or talk about my dream girl in Brooklyn.

Brooklyn was known for fine women, but my high school dream girl had a boyfriend. I really could have been involved with more girls, but I was just too shy. Sometimes I wonder if I missed out or was it simply not meant to be. I was not a good student. Overall, I was a C average student. I'd take an elective in a heartbeat to get around the tough subjects. I probably would have done a lot better, but I started singing in fashion shows and plays while in school. The early years of marijuana use didn't prompt me to study more either. My interest with girls was definitely on the rise. So there I was, this shy kid, being very active in church and in high school, getting high regularly and constantly thinking about girls.

Years later, all that mattered in my life was sex, drugs, and rock & roll. Yes, the cliché was true; at least it was for me. I've been working since I was fourteen. Once you get a taste of what it takes to make money, how to survive, and how to satisfy your own desires, you would be a fool not to continue earning for self. I heard someone say that the first law of nature is the preservation of self. Always having a little something is better than having nothing at all. I've always had the skill to talk with the best of them; I just had to work up to it. If you put me in a boardroom for twenty minutes, I would find a way to make good conversation even if I didn't know the daily agenda.

It is amazing how a junkie or druggie will always find a way out of no-way to get some money to feed his habit or to simply BS people and try to impress them. Many people that know me to some degree would tell me that I have never had a problem getting a job. The main difference from the old me to the current me is that I would use manipulation for selfish motives, and today I use my assertive, verbal skills for constructive purposes.

I was a force to be reckoned with on many occasions. I am living proof that drugs will make you a different person...period. I was so screwed up in my thinking; I took getting high beyond the limits of reason. Once, I went out with a girl and drank so much it was ridiculous. We went back to my place and put a nightcap on the nightcap. We smoked weed, probably laced it with cocaine or crack. We snorted blow. It got to a point where the evening was about the drugs, not the girl, and not me. Looking at things more realistically, the evening was about how much drugs I can do and what I can do to her with that much in my system. At one point, she felt that she had to throw up. I told her to go ahead and throw up, but I stood directly behind her, and kept engaging her sexually as she tried to relieve herself, finally she said, "Forget it; I can't throw up like that. I'll throw up later."

On a different occasion with someone else, I was so high I could hardly move. I do not know where the money came from, but I just kept going—smoking, snorting, drinking, even when it made me physically sick; I couldn't get enough. I often displayed this side of myself. Most people hang around peers because they share a common bond. The bond could be salary, profession, residence or recreation, but usually there is a bond that ties people together. Some of my friends were astonished by my consumption of drugs and alcohol when I chose to drink.

Once, a friend asked my girlfriend, "Does Charles realize that he's doing everything?" My stash was crack or base, but everyone else was either snorting cocaine, smoking weed, smoking cocaine-laced weed, or cocaine-laced cigarettes, and I did it all. As I think back, it was embarrassing, but that didn't stop me. Sixty percent of my paycheck never lasted longer than twenty-four hours, and it wouldn't matter how much money I made. I actually had to bring home over a thousand dollars weekly in order for that not to be the case. One payday I sat on the couch comatose.

I had one of those drug-crazed evenings of back-to-back getting high. They say some people drink like a fish, referring to alcohol. Well, I was the bottomless pit of smoking crack (King of the Woolahs). A woolah is a hollowed out cigar refilled with marijuana and crack. If powder cocaine is used on a joint it is laced. My heart was racing. My girl took a look at me and said; "You're not feeling too good, are you?" I shook my head no.

It was about two maybe three in the morning and because of my ignorance, I caused her to go outside to the store to get some orange juice. She volunteered without asking, but I still feel that I put her at risk. At that time, in the morning anything could have happened to her. Even if you are from the 'hood, people will lurk in the shadows and catch you. She returned from the store with the juice and I started to come down. What a difference the real vitamin C can make.

When I was getting high, everything else was secondary, including sex. Without going into great detail, and with and without a magazine of choice, I put my imagination to work. I was rarely interested in my girlfriend's interest during those years. I lived a self-centered life with an insatiable appetite for what interested me. I am still working on having control and balance to my life. If my body had a voice of its own, I bet there would have been plenty of arguing. I abused myself so much. I think about how I was getting high and being dehydrated, the effects on my skin, my lungs, my mouth and tongue. What was I thinking? My lack of good hygiene was another embarrassing aspect during my life of drug addiction. It is a wonder that I have not suffered more physical or health-related issues. I put myself through years and years of abuse. There is a price to pay and I am sure in recent years, I was in the paying zone.

There was only one time that I actually played the field to the fullest. I dated a young lady for about five years. We decided to move to a nicer neighborhood. We saved and made all the needed arrangements to move. I was still using heavily. In fact, one day I wanted to take some of the money we were saving so I could get high. I didn't want much, just twenty or thirty dollars, and she bitched with a smart comment. I got up, ran after her and grabbed her by the collar. She knew me, but I had never done anything like that before. She was scared to death.

My mom called my dad, to try to get me to calm down. I know I was not supposed to use the money, but that was why I asked her. I realize, after the fact, that I was not being rational even though she was being a smart ass, and she was intentionally doing it in front of my mother to embarrass me. After that incident, we got our place, and left the past behind us. I made all the arrangements to get our furniture and personal belongings moved. Finally, we got our place, moved in, and after a few months, she told me that she thought I needed to leave.

I wanted to blow up on her, but I sucked it in and figured I would eventually get my revenge. I started working in Somerville,

New Jersey, and just fumbling around from job to job. Every now and then, I would come back to New York City and try to stop by to see my ex, hoping to score. I guess she got me back for trying to choke her out. I moved back in with my mom and continued to see my ex-girl when I could, but I also kept my dating options open. I started seeing a co-worker where I worked for a music production company, and several others, like the financial aid officer from the technical school I attended. She thought I was so cute. I found out that she lived near my mom, so I paid her a visit one Sunday. I was hoping to extend that into a decent relationship. She was young and attractive; she had her own apartment, and she liked me. The sad thing about that period in my life was that my hygiene was up and down. I had good and bad days.

When I visited the financial aid officer, it was a bad day. I barely washed up and I didn't have clean clothes, which was very embarrassing. I was alone with her on a Sunday afternoon, and we were about to get intimate and I had on dirty underclothes and outer clothes. I didn't represent that day. It was a humiliating experience of which I brought on myself. I never saw her again. I was still trying to get revenge on my ex-girlfriend. In addition to everything that I was going through, I still had to keep my habit up and conceal it from those that didn't know how bad I was strung out. I later met an ex-high school sweetheart, and there were a couple of others. I didn't have sex with all of them, but that was how I got my revenge.

When it came to playing the field, which I didn't do very often, I was never caught. The only thing about playing the field is whether you are caught or not, you have to be able to live with yourself. There is a saying that some things you are supposed to take to your grave with you. I think it is true even if it is because of Alzheimer's.

It was very difficult for me to learn from my experiences during those years. First, it was because I was still getting high all the time. That meant I still had to sort through the cloudy moments and retain whatever my brain could comprehend. Then, I guess one of the final lessons would be that since the pain was not as bad, I could really try to move on without so much remorse or heartache.

I distinctly remember living in the Bronx, going through some crazy times. I lived on Gerard Avenue and 157th Street, right behind Yankee Stadium, and right next to the #4 train. It was a predominantly Latino neighborhood. Blacks and Latinos primarily sold weed on the corners, and cocaine and dope seemed to have been controlled by Latinos solely. I was smoking so much crack it was pathetic. By this time my daughter and her mother had moved, I was still jamming with the band, but I just stayed jacked up.

One day, my sister whom is eleven years younger than I am, decided to tell me about myself. I couldn't believe she wanted to put me in check.

5/31/84

Dear Charles,

I know I'm not your mother nor your father but I'm your sister and I care. It's hurting me to see what you are doing to yourself. I love you and I want you to be around long. Charles you don't know how much your putting mom threw. At night she cry today she was crying. It's hurting mom to see you this way. Your getting thinner and starting to look bad. You forgetting all about the love ones. I don't know how you and Charlene are but I do no she loves you and your hurting her. She's a very nice person and you just might lose her. Charles get your self together go back to the way you were. I love you and I'm here but if you don't try or get some kind of help then I don't want to be bother with you and I mean it.

Love
Morgan

This is what she wrote:

May 31st, 1986

Dear Charles

I know I'm no your mother nor your father but I'm your sister and I care. It's hurting me to see what you are doing to yourself. I love you and I want you to be around long. Charles you don't know how much your putting mom threw. At night she cry today she was crying. It's hurting mom to see you this way.

You're getting thinner and starting to look bad. You're forgetting all about your love ones. I don't know how you and Charlene are but I do no she loves you and you're hurting her. She's a very nice person and you just might lose her. Charles get yourself together go back to the way you were. I love you and I'm here, but if you don't try or get some kind of help then I don't want to be bothered with you and I mean it.

Love

Monique Medina

Out of all the drugs I consumed, I never used intravenous drugs. Needles could never be my style. Besides that, I was doing enough of everything else anyway. Drinking alcohol or beer was child's play to me. I smoked weed, angel dust, took blotter, mescaline, yellow jackets, speed, sniffed coke, smoked coke, sniffed speed balls, laced cigarettes with coke, laced marijuana with cooked and powdered coke. If I couldn't get any of my favorites, then I would resort to the child's play category of drinking beer or liquor. I am damn lucky to have a brain.

Breaking up and getting together is just a part of life, whether drugs are involved or not. I guess the main lesson for me was to acknowledge that I needed to think straight and the only way to do that was to get off drugs. I would bet that was one of the biggest challenges I've ever had in life.

We all will need someone or something at some point or time...I need God, how about you?

—C. Cary

Trueality Enterprises

Chapter 14

LOCKDOWN

As a teen growing up, Harlem had its advantages and disadvantages, and I experienced a good amount of both. I remember after I started buying my own weed, I would roll up, and sometimes stick a joint behind my ear. One day a cop drove by and told me to take it from behind my ear, because I didn't have a license for it. That scared the crap out of me, but it also sent me mixed messages. It basically told me, it's ok to do drugs, just do not let anybody know and do not get caught.

I was first exposed to drugs when I was maybe seven or eight years old. My step-dad would get an album cover and clean an ounce or a half-ounce of weed, roll it up and get blitzed. I didn't know what it was until I got a little older, but I hated the smell and I vowed to never ever smoke it. Fast forward six or seven years, when my brother came home from prison, he would ask me if I wanted to spend the weekend with him. You know I wanted to hang out with my brother. There were all of these fine sister's around and we would smoke weed. I loved being away from the nest so that I could get a little dirt up under my nails.

I was not able to go every weekend, but when I had the opportunity, I was out! By the time I was 13 and in the 8th grade, I was pretty game for anything. The only thing that scared me was

LSD. A lot of people were bugging out over LSD. While in the 8th grade our senior class went to Washington D.C., my hometown. All of the boys got together and decided to get high. We chipped in and bought some weed and some *Boone's Farm* wine. It was my first attempt at getting high independently. As I recall there was at least a half dozen of us chugging on the wine and slobbering all over the joints because we were using cherry flavored *Bambu* rolling paper. We stood in between all of the buses where they dropped us off and got high. I felt independent, but I do not remember if I felt a buzz.

It was just a few mere years afterwards, I'd be buying weed for Pete and he would occasionally buy weed for me. Was he setting me up or just paying for the convenience? Those were very tense times between my stepfather and me. His mother and father died, and he felt quite alone. He couldn't read and blamed others for his shortcomings. Many of these things were not clear at the time. He would boast and bark at anything for seemingly no reason at all. I hated him at certain points in my life. He wanted to challenge me because he couldn't reach me and I wouldn't side with him just because. He meant well, but he just didn't know the proper way to go about it.

He told me a few things that I will always remember and I will always appreciate. The first thing was to always be observant of my surroundings. The second was, that if I ever found out that I couldn't look at myself in the mirror, there was a problem. The first piece of advice came in handy. The second piece of advice took a couple of decades before I'd realize what was happening to me.

The first time I went to jail I was about twenty-nine years old. I stopped to see my cousin; he was selling whatever you needed. I can't forget this, not just because it was my first jail visit, but also because the Knicks and the Bulls were playing. It was a big game with Michael Jordan. My friend Phil and I stopped by to pick up some cocaine. A few of my cousin's friends were there. We were just sitting around talking mess. We heard a knock on the door; I think some guy wanted to buy something with short money but he was turned away. A few minutes later another knock came. It was the police. They asked if they could come in because of a disturbance being reported so after about a minute, we let them in.

Everything was fine until Officer Kilroy saw the triple beam scale in the kitchen. The scale had a little residual powder on it too. He demanded that nobody move. A few moments later they said we were all under arrest. When they knocked on the door the first time I guess my cousin must have had a bad feeling of something. He had run into the bedroom to hide his gun, and he said he poured water into a big bag of cocaine. The police found some drugs, paraphernalia, and eventually the gun..

The police had us, but the charges were going to stick on the owner of the apartment. We were all handcuffed and marched down into police cars driven away to face our destiny. We all were embarrassed by what happened but my cousin; Diamond Dave

took it extra hard. He always came across like a Big Willie type.

Now, he was busted! We were adults, but as kids we use to play in

that apartment so much. 80 East 110th Street, I loved visiting as a

kid, but now I was a grown man. My friend Phil was a short

brother and probably the most problematic of all of us. I know he

was scared, in fact I do not think I saw too much of him once the

situation totally unfolded.

One brother, I think his name was John, he had literally just

come home from prison off a rape charge, and the other guy was

just hanging out. Phil and I were coming from work, and of course

my cousin was the one that the cops would try to pin everything

on. We didn't know it at the time, but they really didn't have a

case. Their evidence stood as follows: a gun that didn't work,

drugs that didn't amount to anything substantial and there were not

any drugs being used. But, they hadn't found any drugs on us

during their search. It probably was a waste of time. David had the

biggest problem because he had a criminal record. I was coming

from work dressed in a nice suit and tie, and I couldn't believe it. I

didn't even have a chance to get high. That thought stay in my

mind. I didn't get a chance to smoke a joint!

Before we went to Central Booking, we landed in a local

precinct. In fact, I had a bag of weed on me. The cop flushed it

down the toilet. I made my one phone call and it was hard calling

my mother with news like this. I was twenty-nine years old, living on my own and I was still scared to make the call. I had to tell my mother the short version of the story. I went to my cousin's house and was locked up. I knew it would upset her, but it had to be done. Mom was used to my brother getting into all sorts of trouble, but not me. I never had a cop put his hands on me. My brother had been to jail and prison. This was all new to me and I didn't want to get used to it. I wanted my cake and I wanted to eat it too. I felt that I could do my dirt and I should be able to get away with it. I spent the night in a jail cell.

We did have a chance at getting a store run. That was before they took our personal belongings. The officers obviously could have been nasty about it but I was grateful they weren't. I had just gotten paid, (like the song says it was Friday night and I had about two hundred and fifty to three hundred dollars in my pocket). The money felt like it was burning a hole in my leg, not my pocket. It was amazing for me to have that much money for more than two or three hours. Normally, one third of that money would have been smoked, snorted and swallowed within two to three hours after getting off of work. The store run was the only highlight of the evening.. I bought a couple of Snickers and a pack of Newport cigarettes. I was sucking those Newport's down fast because I hadn't smoked a joint, or drank anything. We finally got to Central Booking, only to be humiliated by some muscle bound cop that thought he was the judge and the jury.

He wanted to know why I had a ponytail. One guy was so embarrassed he didn't even have on underwear; he had fabric wrapped around his butt. The man went down the line inmate by inmate, just trying to break us down and challenge us. We finally went to the bullpen. As I said before, my cousin had lots of experience being locked up just like my brother did. David gave me a quick lesson in jailhouse etiquette telling me not to give away cigarettes and not to let people play me for my goods.

I understood all of that; I just was not planning on being there too long. My cousin started telling people that we were ready to set it off up in bullpen, and if anybody wanted to get busy all they had to do was step. He had the nerve to tell them I was a black belt and wouldn't think twice about breaking bones. He took me by surprise but I understood his rationale for doing this.

The cops brought a couple of guys in that had beef with each other and man did they get that place going. They started rolling up in that piece like it was a rehearsal. This little guy started banging this guy's head into the bars like he was playing timbales. I mean the entire experience was a little nerve racking. They gave us bologna and cheese to eat. They also served tea with lots of Thorazine. I guessed they wanted to keep us mellow (Thorazine is probably considered a standard beverage for an upscale joint like central booking). The tormenting part about it was sitting around thinking the worst would happen, and just not knowing if it would.

The next day we'd face the judge. We were shuttled downtown to 80 Centre Street, so that we could all be arraigned one by one. They called Phil before me. He looked nervous; his father met him in court. When they called my name, I could taste freedom. I stood before the judge and the prosecuting attorney started talking about how I was a risk, because I went AWOL and had all of these robberies on my record. My lawyer immediately asked me why I hadn't told him. I was shocked; I didn't know what that other lawyer was talking about. The funny thing was whomever she was talking about had my name, birthday, place of birth and everything. I had to go back to a holding cell. I couldn't believe what I was hearing.

The entire weekend I was absolutely frazzled. I kept lying to myself, over and over. I had made up my mind that there would be no more drugs in my life. Meanwhile, my lawyer needed to verify my credentials. They requested information f to verify the facts. I must have waited for another fifteen minutes before coming back out to face the judge, although it seemed much longer. I thought my clean-cut look would bail me out. I do not know how much it worked for me though. I hadn't showered or shaved for two days. I also began to expect the worst. I was not sure if they would get a more positive ID than what they already had presented to the court. I kept thinking that I was on my way to Rikers Island. They could only get a picture via fax, and you know a fax machine won't do a beauty queen any justice. The fax finally came and thank God, you could tell the guy that was using my name, didn't look anything like me. There was no comparison. Finally, they let me go. All I had to do was make my upcoming court appearances for the case.

I went back to the holding cell with the other guys. I got my personal effects and we all stood outside for a few minutes. My partner and I were the only individuals with cash, remember we had just got paid. I bought hot dogs for everybody. I went Uptown and the first thing I did was buy a half gram of crack to get high. My money would only last two or three days. I was back to my daily routine.. I had not learned my lesson.

The next time I got caught up, I was trying to make a purchase in Washington Heights. Actually, it started when I ran into one of my partners from around the way. Hassan was a street hustler. Some days he would be washing cars, and other days he might be selling merchandise that he found or stole. I believe all people possess good and bad traits. Especially those in the streets, who do not receive credit for the good they possess. I guess you do have to catch them on a good day, but that does not stop it from being true. Hassan and his girl, Jane, would see me going to and from work or see me with my children. They may have thought that I was the cool working guy from the neighborhood, but they knew I got high. With that being the case, they didn't stop them from asking me for change from time to time. It was totally perplexing to me that I had the same problem that they had. I would come home and change clothes, go out and buy drugs

every single day.

Jane disappeared one day and I didn't see her for a long

time. I later found out that she was hospitalized, and died from

AIDS. It was pretty safe to say, most of us that knew her and

Hasaan knew that he probably contracted the virus also. One day

when the neighborhood seemed to be pretty dry, I mean I couldn't

find any drugs anywhere. I saw Hassan, and he told me that he

knew of a place. I decided to go with him. The first drug spot we

went to, well let's just say that that spot was a bust. In fact there

was this big cop right behind us as we came out of the building. He

stopped us and questioned us but to no avail we didn't have

anything on us. As we continued our quest for the goods, we found

ourselves on Amsterdam Avenue.

We went up to the sixth floor. We got what we went there

for. I was pleasantly surprised. On the way downstairs Hassan said,

"Wait!" He heard something. I thought he was bugging, maybe

even trying to scam me. His streetwise insight was on point. It was

kind of like how Spiderman says, "My spidey senses are tingling."

I waited for a couple of minutes and became impatient. I've always

considered myself different/special. I know that I am, but the thing

is, if you are not living according to the plan that God has laid out

for you, then you may not have the opportunity to tap into that

special something. So here I am on the staircase, in this building where every floor has one or two apartments out of 6 that sells drugs.

I grew impatient trying to wait out the cop on the first floor. I felt like I could walk by the cops and just walk out of the door. I also felt that because I worked as a white-collar worker and my neck tie reflected as such, I would not be questioned. I figured I'd bluff the cop when he approached me but when he challenged me, I gave in. He wanted me to prove that I had a reason to be in the building. I was arrested, went to jail and Hassan got away.

My family was waiting for me to come home with a loaf of bread and that never happened. I was finger printed, and put on ice. Once again I didn't know what to expect. I kept thinking about where I could stash the cocaine I had on me. I knew that if they did a strip search, I was done. The cop that followed us earlier was processing whoever got arrested. He kept telling the other guys that there would be a strip search. One guy must have been really afraid, because he just kept nervously running his mouth. He would ask one question after another.

I had drugs on me, and New York's Finest didn't find it. I was ready to throw it away, but was not a trash can in the jail cell. I thought of every possible scenario and I just prayed that they didn't find the drugs. They ran a check on me and came up with nothing. After a couple of hours they let me go. I was so happy; I couldn't wait to get home. Sad to say as soon as I got home I explained what had happened to me. My girl was thoroughly disgusted. All I kept thinking was I was safe and as soon as she shut up, I could go and get high. I didn't realize how sick I was. Just the thought of those times still bring back such a realistic feeling of dissatisfaction and despair.

Something about living through a drug induced state of mind can be very scary. The thought of things I've done have stayed with me and from time to time seems to haunt me. Although it has been several years since I've had a drink or used drugs, it seems certain thought awaken a very realistic sensation within me. I can almost taste the smoke coming out of my mind, or I can feel the sensation of being in suspended animation over getting more drugs. It's sick.

These were some crucial times when God was trying to get my attention and I didn't realize what was happening to me or around me. In church we are taught that we should raise a child as he or she should grow and those ways should never depart from them. I was so saturated with guilt, filth, and sin that I didn't realize what was happening. I thank God that his mercy was extended to a lowly sinner like me. I can't imagine if it hadn't been?

Chapter 15

BROTHERS

I always loved my brother and no matter what I always will. When he was locked up on Rikers Island I use to write these sloppy letters to him from time to time, because I loved him and missed him so much. When he came home he found a way of letting me know how much those letters meant to him. They broke him down inside, because I guess he realized I was trying to be like him, and I didn't know what to expect from the big ole world we lived in.

There are so many feelings and emotions I have when it comes to describing my relationship with my brother. I felt that I loved him more than my mother. I would say that I attribute that thought and feeling to the fact that when my mom was fed up with our father she moved on temporarily, so that she could prepare the best life for us as she saw fit. In her absence my brother was the only constant I could identify with. When we lived on Irving Street in D.C., he would come and go and always take a few minutes for his baby brother. He was a real big brother. He'd bring me toys to play with that he found or maybe even gotten from another source. I remember him and my sister Leila trying to teach me how to ride a bike in the basement when I was two or three years old. He tried to teach me how to fight, and how to drive a car describing it on a piece of paper. Can you imagine learning how to drive from

pencil and paper?

After my Mother came back to get me from my Father, my young mind was on cloud 50. I was going to the liquor store with my dad one day, and who did I see walking down the street towards us…my senses said one thing, but my conscious mind said…I am not sure. It was my mother, my sister, and my brother. When I actually realized it was my brother, I broke away from my father and ran as fast as I could to my brother and dove right into his arms! You could hear the orchestrated music playing just like in a big movie production. Oh my god, I love my brother so much, as I write these words…it takes me right back to Irving Street in Washington, DC. This happened to have been one of those times when my brother had run away from home.

My father couldn't believe it when my mother came back to get me. When she told him that she was here for me, he simply conceded. I guess after all of the years of playing hardball with her, and being mean to mom, he had no fight left. From there we went to my grandmother's house to get me cleaned up, and prepare me for the trip to my new home. My brother helped me get use to things in New York. I learned many of the fundamentals and then some. When we settled in Harlem, we live on 7th Avenue between 146th Street & 147th Street across the street from Esplanade Gardens before it was built. There was a bar on the corner of 146th, a Laundromat next to that, a couple of apartment buildings, and

then a church, then next to the church was a cleaners, and then
our building 2528 7th Avenue #9, on the 5th floor.

Everybody used the Laundromat on the corner. My brother
would start the clothes, then go play with his friends and lose all
track of the time, and get in trouble every time. So I learned how to
wash clothes by default. Then there was the time he took me to
church and started playing basketball in his church clothes and had
to explain how he tore his clothes in church. One of my favorite
stories was how he got a puppy and tried to hide it under the bed
and nobody knew but him and me. My mom was preparing me for
a recital in church and she kept hearing a whimpering as she tied
my necktie (yeah, mom was good like that she taught me how to
tie a tie. It was not a Windsor knot, but it got the job done.
Anyway, she told me to stop making that noise, and I said "I am
not making noise". The next time the dog whimpered, she said
"what is that then?" I told her it was our dog…She was scared to
death for about 5 seconds until I showed her it was a puppy. I
almost pissed my pants laughing. My brother was in trouble again
and had to get rid of the puppy. He had to get rid of a nice green
ten-speed bike also, as I remember.

In my opinion nothing penetrates true sibling love. Not
pain, not distance, not crime, I mean absolutely nothing. Once
there was a time when he just made curfew by literally one minute.
I was so happy for him because the boy was a chronic trouble
magnet. We would stay up and play with G.I. Joes or watch TV

until the sun came up. *Reel Camp* was our favorite late night

show. This one night in particular, practically the whole house was

celebrating him not being in trouble again. He and I went into our

room and he started telling me about this fight he had with a guy

who thought he could beat him. My brother must have busted him

up. He started to describe the fight blow by blow, and as he is

showing me in real time how he dropped a fast wicked uppercut on

the other boy; I looked directly into the path of his swinging fist.

Bam! He busted my left eye wide open. There was blood all over

the place. I was screaming in pain at first, then my mother and Pete

came running in the room screaming. He tried to cover my mouth

to muffle the sound before they came in, but it was too late and too

loud.

About a minute later Pete made him get out. Initially I was

crying because of the punch, and it was one of those long cries

where you feel like you are running out of air in between each

gasp. You can't talk, because you are trying to control your

breathing and crying. I was not able to tell them that it was an

accident. I was no longer hurt by the pain of the punch; my brother

being made to leave hurt me. I would have gladly taken a punch to

the other eye if I could just have my brother stay. My eye took

about a month to heal, with a ton of cocoa butter. It would take my

heart so much longer to heal.

My horizons were about to be shaken. When I was thirteen

my brother introduced me to the Islamic faith. He wanted me to be able to take care of myself and I think by now he would be pleased. He meant, and still means so much to me. When he introduced me to Islam - I definitely wanted to learn more about it. The realization that Columbus couldn't discover a land where people have already settled began to open my mind. During my thirteenth and fourteenth year I was beginning to be stretched mentally and didn't even realize it. Learning how black people were the first known people on the planet, and how we are actually a majority versus a minority really started to build an inner pride. .

Studying The Book of Life would take some getting used to. I didn't have the discipline for it but I had a mentor in my brother, and he would see to it that I would learn. I am a Christian today, but I will always have respect for Islam. I would visit my brother in the Bronx on the weekends and smoke reefer, absorb the five percent culture, and really begin to find myself. I had adopted the name Master because that was my degree (my age). M is the thirteenth letter of the alphabet, and I had to be able to understand what my name meant and break it down upon request.

Every letter of the alphabet has a word associated to it, and as it is define there is a deeper meaning to the word itself, and a deeper meaning to the discussion. For example, my name is Charles if I break it down in the alphabet you would get: C –He-Allah-Rule-Love-Equality-Self. So imagine how each discussion can have a prolonged and intense purpose or meaning. This was also a good way to communicate when using abbreviations.

We would also have rallies, study, and go to Parliaments.. The Book of Life was the equivalent to the Torah, or the Bible. The Five- Percent Nation seemed to be comprised of many offenders and ex-offenders that would really like to do the right thing, but it was a huge achievement to accomplish. It was about saving the babies and helping black people become conscious.

It was the 70's and a lot of brothers were messing up. They were not only getting high, but also they were selling drugs and still doing stick-ups. Now, I do not have proof of any specific situation, but if you are from the street you know what goes on around you. I was always pretty observant. Let it be known there was a lot of good also. The gods, as they are called, would have meetings about the direction they wanted to go in. My brother Kyleke, as he was now called was very instrumental in advocating for events on behalf of the nation. There was always a rally of some sort. The purpose was to teach the young gods and the babies. They did try to educate, feed, and give the young brothers something to do even if they weren't doing the right thing all the time. There were a lot of agendas. I was never in the hierarchy or anything, but my brother was.

He would help by organizing trips and being a steward over a community location in the Bronx so that the youth would have a place to study after school. I know that out of the five boroughs in New York, there was pretty good communication, but when my brother disappeared nobody knew anything. I remember reading about the history of the 5 Percent Nation on the Internet. The article was titled "The BOMB (The Greatest Story Never Told)" by Beloved Allah. *Another event that further illustrates that the forces that killed Allah were alive and active in the Bronx took place in 1976. A very sincere God by the name of Kyleek had acquired use of the local manpower office for use of the Gods and Earths in the community to hold classes in martial arts, sewing, etc.... He had the keys to the building and was responsible for opening it up every day, which he did faithfully. One day he didn't show up to open the building and he hasn't been heard from since.*

This all that was said or known about my brother, the activist, the father, the son, the man that cared about young life and it's development in the inner city.

There were no hospital records, police reports, arrest records or anything suspicious to go on. I used to go to the school in Mecca (Manhattan) and speak to the gods about my brother's whereabouts, but to no avail. After a while I stopped going by. It seemed almost impossible that out of all the people he introduced me to; everyone I spoke with knew nothing. I even found out many years later that my mother spent money on private detectives and they came up empty. There was this one cop my mom knew who claimed that my brother was in Sing Sing or Attica, but was in solitary with no visitors because he had no respect for authority

but that was in the eighties.

My brother had three Earth's (spouses) and none of them said they knew anything concrete. Some of his women were much newer to the ways of the nation than others. At this time his latest Earth was Miasia; I used to spend the weekends at her crib. She had five sisters and a brother, but only three of the sisters hung out with us on the weekends, and we never saw her brother. I went to high school with one of her sisters and boy was that an odd situation. I remember her coming up to me asking me who I am and saying that her sister is dating my brother. At the time we were in a brand new high school, with hundreds of kids around us on 8 out of 10 floors all day, and when she came up to me, I was thinking ok so now what? Then slowly but surely I became intrigued with the idea of knowing that my brother and I were linked to sisters. It seemed like we were supposed to automatically go out; it eventually happened, but initially I had no interest.

When we first started dating we would just make out in the subway station at her stop and that is as far as we went. I think she came over to visit once. I was all goofy and didn't know what to do with myself. The weekends in the Bronx at her sister's house were priceless though. We always had a blast, playing music, getting high, getting the munchies and pigging out. Pardon the pun but we didn't eat pork. We were really close, the entire clan. We'd take pictures and just party. The entire crew would often spend the night there in the Bronx at Miasia's house. We partied so much; we never studied like we were supposed to.

Diana and I broke up at the end of the school year and believe it or not, it broke my heart. I asked her what I did but she never told me. (It was a stinging and very disappointing feeling to find out that I was not wanted. Those early rejections and let downs, set the pace of how I played the dating game. They determined how much I would reveal my feelings for a woman. If I would be the first to say things like, I love you, and processing the lingering pain that led into the next relationship.

After a while Kyleke didn't want me to spend the night, having fun getting high all the time. He seemed to become much more serious. I do not know if it was because I was not being a leader or because I just hung out with a bunch of women. I often wonder if it could have even had something to do with his eventual disappearance. It seemed as though he couldn't spend time with me because he was out wheeling and dealing almost of the time. He finally told me to stop getting high so much. I felt something was going on, but I just didn't know what it was. It was his expression and his mood that had changed. He was always on the go

I found it difficult to trust anyone, although the next year, I would date someone else. The reality of my circumstances was that I was a sensitive and emotional person, and being male it seemed odd because it was always implied that guys don't deal with sensitivity.

It was my junior year and her name was Rina- although she seemed to be caught up on some guy in Job Core. We went out a few times, and got physical a few times too. After dating for a while she told me about her Job Core friend and said that we couldn't be super serious…too late…I had already gotten attached.

The funny thing about that situation was that she didn't wait for Mr. Job Core, she had a baby with someone else and life went on. I didn't stay upset about it. Life turns out the way it's supposed to. Around that time I was singing a lot. Soon I would be given my first solo with the MLK Ensemble. I thought that I was on my way.

At this time my brother was M.I.A. for about a year or two. I was really missing him. I had a few girlfriends that I wanted him to meet as I was maturing. I guess I wanted brotherly advice and opinions as the years went on. When my brother and I were kids we use to talk about how it would be when we grew up. We would have homes and cars near one another. Those things never happened. I remember one of the last things he said to me, "Do not think when you die, I'll see you in heaven and all that. When you are dead, you are dead, that's all". Kyleke seemed to have such a pissed off outlook on life. After his disappearance I didn't hang out with many people from the Five Percent inner circle only Miasia and her sisters and that was once in a while.

How he disappeared is still a mystery. My brother's Earth, Roshamella called and asked had I seen my brother. I immediately said no, and I was not sure what to think. The thought crossed my mind that I needed to look for him, but I didn't know where to start or what to do. Roshamella said that in the past my brother would spend time with the other Earths and once he was in Connecticut for a while without letting her know, but he came home. The story is that Roshamella and my brother lived in the Bronx and had a rent party. They moved all of the furniture to the roof, so that they would have space for their guests I do not know how successful the party was, but after the party my brother was bringing the furniture back in the house and at some point he disappeared.

I do not know if he finished bringing the furniture back in the house or not, but that was the last time she said she saw him. As I write this I am thinking about the fact that the New York City Police Department seemed to be coming down on the Five Percent Nation because at the time they were organized and gathering momentum with all of their initiatives. So my question is, since he was part of their problem did they have anything to do with his disappearance to create a satisfactory solution for the higher ups of New York's Finest? All of his other Earth's had not seen him and didn't know where he could have been. My brother was the one sibling that I could communicate with as far back as I could remember. I felt I should have done more to find out what happened to him. I wanted to keep going by the school when I was younger, but I started to think that if I became a nuisance then somebody might try to get rid of me too.

Now that introduces the second theory. My brother's friend Kamel, were together all the time. I find it nearly impossible that Kamel didn't have any idea about what could have happened. When you saw Kyleke, you saw Kamel that's how close they were. It was like Batman & Robin. The road to achievement does not wind the same way for everyone. So I wonder if my brother and his cut partner Kamel got a package and things go wrong, or did my brother get a package on his own and things went wrong?

If that happened then somebody would have to pay up in one way or another. In other words, if my theory was correct and I kept coming around someone at the school did know something about what happened to my brother. I could have been seen as a threat and expendable. From time to time, I'd run into some of the brothers that I met during the 70's. They would be glad to see me, but still had no idea what happened to my brother.

When I was in treatment at Samaritan Village for my drug problem I spoke to a couple of guys from the lower eastside about my brother. They told me that they knew someone fitting that description from the area. I can't explain it, but I never investigated it. It seems that my brother's disappearance has given me an opportunity to grow up on my own. I have had to take my bumps and bruises without a physical guardian angel. Maybe I have had a spiritual guardian angel, and I have been blind to its

presence. There have not been many days since 1974 that I do not

think about Anthony Lewis Smith A.K.A. Kyleke Allah. He'll

always be with me, even if it is in spirit. I do feel that I will find

out about his whereabouts one day, but until that day may God and

Holy Ghost fill me enough to redirect the path that my nephew

strives on, if it is the Lord's will.

*Friends can be closer than brothers, but there's always an
exception to the rule.*

—*C. Cary*

Chapter 16

MR. MUSIC

During that summer of 1979, I felt like music was calling my name. At this time, I had been performing for about five years with the MLK Ensemble. I was the seasoned tenor and my boy Eddie had recently joined; we sang together along with Darryl Johnson. We called ourselves the Three Scorpio Tenors). The original ensemble members had moved on for one reason or another. Eddie and I were trying to recruit Paul who had left the group and went on to a much more promising music career. We needed him to play piano for us. Eddie and I loved music and decided to audition in a contest held by the Institute for New Cinema Arts; Ossie Davis was the President at that time.

The company was based in midtown Manhattan, but the actual performance would take place at Grant's Tomb. We decided the songs that we wanted to sing were "Always and Forever" by Heatwave and *Chocolate Girl* by The Whispers. We tried to get George to play for us, but he wouldn't. George was our coordinator for the MLK movement.

Eddie and I were finally able to convince Paul Lawrence to play for us. We made it to the semi-finals. There were soloists, bands, and a wide variety of performers. I was nervous, but ready. We did our songs; it was nice to put it to you plainly. We didn't go any further than the semifinals. The group that won was Climax. I would run into some of their members later. Teddy Riley was

the keyboard player and Greg Birch was the drummer for Climax.

I will always be in love with music. It has been a part of my

life for as long as I can remember. I have probably sung at every

church in New York City, some in Philly, and a few in Delaware,

DC and New Jersey. Even through the years drug use, music has

always been there for me. It would have been nice if it was

therapeutic, but it was not. Drugging has been more hypnotic than

anything. Now that I think about it, I could have treated my music

better. For almost forty years I've been doing this and I still love it.

At one time, I took off five years only to come back with such a

deeper desire and respect for it. I couldn't help it; music was

calling me. *To thine own self be true.*

My getting high was like breathing air. It was something

that I had to do and it went with singing and performing.

There are times when a song strikes a chord in me. I mean

it just, sets off a thirst and a rush of memories. It's a feeling so

hard to explain. Performing in front of people, seeing their faces

light up, doing the song just like the original artist elated me. The

feeling of being onstage was the ultimate high. That same feeling

is apparent when I am writing or just talking to people that I have

something in common with learning from each other and sharing

information and opinions, it's absolutely great!

What a perfect life-style for a hypocrite. Music was sort of

floating in the background. I'd enjoy it on the weekends but that was it. I sang to records I liked, but I was not sure of what to do. A few years later I decided that I needed to be serious about it. I started buying the music papers like *Backstage, Show Business,* and *The Village Voice* to get an idea of what was going on in the business. After getting caught up on what was happening I went on many auditions and cattle calls. It was a very good experience. Those auditions kept me in shape, they kept me abreast of what was going on in the industry and it was a great confidence booster.

In our church circle there were some would be celebrities in the ranks. Of all of our friends, Freddie Jackson and Paul Lawrence made a mark in the industry for quite some time. We all were pretty close. We were from different churches in the Harlem area. Collectively we were a very good assortment of talented voices, and musicians. Paul Lawrence came out of White Rock Baptist on 127th street. Freddie Jackson was from a church on Lenox Avenue. I think it was Mt. Olivet. Their group started out from the White Rock Youth Choir, then they became a Paul Lawrence Jones Ensemble, then a few changes in personnel, and they were PLJ. I checked the group out at many showcases and performances in the New York City area. I was a friend, I was a groupie, and I was a sponge because I sucked it all up. It was like class for me, the showcases, the studio sessions man, you couldn't get a better education. Many times you didn't have to ask questions. All you had to do was listen, learn, and remain a student of the game

I do not know if Paul ever realized how much his career educated me. By the time they had set up a few showcases and dropped a good demo, it seemed that recording executives were only interested in Freddie and Lawrence. I guess Freddie for his vocal talent and stage presence and Lawrence for his attributes as a writer, singer, and arranger. I sat in on many of their sessions and had a really good time while learning. Before they blew up, we'd all hang out on a pretty frequent basis and smoke weed or whatever. One day Lawrence just stopped getting high. Gene, Tracy, Darlene, Donna, Val, and I were sort of surprised. Then seemingly not to long after that Freddie got his deal, things were really working out for them. A few years later I was not doing so well because of my drug addiction. I saw Lawrence driving down 7th Avenue right through Harlem in his new Jaguar. I flagged him down and we talked for a few minutes before he was on his way.

Lawrence went on to work with people like Evelyn King, Lilo Thomas, Kashif, and Melba Moore. In fact Melba came down to check out Freddie's showcase. That's how HUSH Productions Capitol picked up Freddie and got him signed to Capitol Records. I really wanted to expand on my musical talents, but that would not happen until a few years down the line.

The group from the choir and ensemble (Gene, Tracy, Darlene, Val, and myself) tried to get a soul / r & b group together once. Think about it, we had all of the components minus the band. We had a few rehearsals and we practiced Heatwave's *Too Hot To*

Handle and *Boogie Nights*. After rehearsals all we could think about was smoking weed. We were back to our normal routine. After we all left high school and began college and getting real jobs, I began exploring deeper with drugs and deeper with music. I relied on some of my earlier experiences with cattle calls and auditions to guide me with music related decisions. I would eventually get my own band.

One Saturday while at my second job some guys walk by with some musical equipment. I stopped them and asked them who they were and where they were going. They rehearsed on the rooftop Saturday and Sunday, from two o'clock to eight o'clock. I asked him did they have a singer and they didn't. I expressed my interest in hearing the band. Darrell, the bass player asked me if I could stop by and test my vocal skills. I was definitely game. I wanted to leave right away and go with them but it was best that I didn't.

I got off work at two o'clock and went right over to 165th Street and Walton Avenue. They were rehearsing on the roof. I went up and told them what songs I knew. There was a full live band set up. Everyone had an instrument in hand, or a cigarette, joint, or a bottle of beer. I do not mean to make it sound like a drug den. That's just the way it was. Frankly, in most music environments that's considered normal.

We tried *Too Hot* by Kool & the Gang. I gave it all I had. I poured my and soul into it and they loved it! I loved it too! The chemistry was set. I became part of the band as the lead singer. The name of the band was F.R.E.E. Over the years, we tried different names: Movin' Heavy and 6 D, but we would always be known as F.R.E.E.

Although it seemed like we rehearsed forever, every Saturday and Sunday from two o'clock to eight o'clock is when it happened until we were tight.. We went through several roster changes. We had an array of musicians, like Joe. Joe would turn his head towards the nearest wall and watch his shadow. I do not know why but it seemed like he was concentrating or keeping his timing by watching the shadow.

Then there was Davy Boy. He was more of a rock style drummer. He had skills, but he just played loud mostly of the time. Davy Boy was a good dude. You could always rely on him. He was on time and he would be ready to play. Paradise on percussion, he would fly in and out. We had James, also known as Gimme Some Roy. I have no clue what that meant.

I was the male lead vocalist. I was still singing in church at the time, so my skills were respectable. Although I must admit the more I played and sang hard, I used drugs harder. We had an array of female vocalists. I believe the first female vocalist was a woman named Ike. She could sing, but she was so damn shy and she never did a gig with us. She was from the neighborhood right there on 165th Street. Then there was Naomi, who was from Brooklyn, and made a few rehearsals but never gigged with us either.

Sunshine came into the group one summer. She was from California and left when the summer was over. Now Coffee was pretty regular. Coffee even gigged with us. She was from Brooklyn and came to the group with Poppa D or Dorian as he was best known. By that time Coffee was in and out and Sunny was the regular. Sunny was the groupie. We found out that she was a trained dancer that could actually sing. When she joined the band she just had not been dancing for a while. Sunny became the lead female vocalist.

The excitement was starting to dwindle down and so were the members. This Puerto Rican kid named DJ Louie Lou wanted to audition and what an audition it was. Louie had that Spanish flavor. He made the drums sing, scream dance and a few more things. We definitely had to have him in the band. He replaced the existing drummer and that was all she wrote. The band was reduced to five core members. We wrote songs, recorded demos, and many times we would make a song on the spot. I would get the forms and send everything to the Library of Congress to copyright the music, or start our bank account. I was serious with it. Although everyone participated on the creative side, we wanted to have a specific sense of direction.

We played all over New York. We played for politicians, we played *The 371 Club, The Celebrity Club, Parkside Plaza, Broadway International, Savoy Manor*, and we even played downtown at a club near Lincoln Center. My mother never liked the band. She felt that they played too loud. Actually she was right in many cases. We never had a soundman and it was almost always rough and dirty.

We were known in the Bronx. GQ's Sabu and Raheem were up the street in The Executive Towers on the Grand Concourse. The band played together for quite a few years. We were a band of brothers. Darryl left for the military, came back, we played a year or two later, and he moved to South Carolina. We didn't hear from him after that. He was a little on the wild side, but damn he was nice on the bass. I would put him up against any bassist and give him a few minutes or give him a day and he would learn the bass line to the song and play it down your throat. EZ D was like that. Ron was more like an academic guitarist.. He started out with that Sunburst Carlo Robelli. He would get some sheet music to understand the essentials of a song or chord structure and after that he would be good. Ron would play lead or rhythm. In fact he told me that Dorian aka Poppa D taught him how to play guitar. We all eventually went our separate ways.

I know one of the fellas may read this book so I might as well admit it right now. Yes, I did date some of our female vocalist, but it was not by design. It happened; I am admitting it so let's move on. I remember Ron would talk about his cousin Carl T. Smith (*The Smooth One*). Carl played keys, and was a music director for *New Edition* in the early years. Carl came around a few times, and we'd try to impress him just because an opportunity may have revealed itself but it never happened. Carl was on a different level. Now if we had a manager or producer we may have yielded different results from our band. Years later, I got with Carl on a solo basis and did shows for him in midtown's Cami Hall and even at The Cotton Club. It was good exposure, and the experience to be around a different caliber of artist in the business.

It seemed as if getting high went with everything I did. I got ripped before a show and tried to mellow down or I wanted to rush through a performance, so that I could reward myself. I got high so much that sometimes it seemed like one big party. I can't tell one time from another time. I use to live on the east side of Manhattan and I had a performance at the Beacon theatre off 73rd street. I remember getting high up until the last minute, rushing out of the house; and I couldn't get a bus because I'd already missed it. I walked from the Eastside to the Westside, sweating and practically running. I finally get there sweating like a pig.

I arrived just in time to start singing. That performance at the Beacon Theater would be one of my most memorable performances. I opened up for *Tavares, The Intruders, The Manhattans, and Harold Melvin & The Blue Notes.* Harold and Co. didn't show up.. I sang a duet, which was really a background part on Whitney Houston's, *Where Do Broken Hearts Go.* I didn't get paid, but it was a milestone, and the moment it was over you know what I did.

I've done sales pretty much all of my life. I worked for DS-Max, a direct sales company that sent me to Acapulco, Mexico. I honestly didn't think that I was going until the day I showed up for work. A limo pulled up and drove us to LaGuardia Airport. I got sloshed on the plane and when I arrived it was just wild to think I was in Mexico. I remember hearing the band practicing thinking to myself how cool it was.

The next day sales people from all over the world got together for a dinner and recognition ceremony. Upon arrival in Acapulco some of the local people sold novelty items, tee shirts, kites, and some of them also tried to sell but I was not going for it. I guess they knew we were from the United States. I went back to the hotel to tell some of my partners from New York about the action on the beach instead, they told me to come on in, close the door, and put a towel down because they had already bought the weed. We rolled blunts and smoked on the terrace. I remembered the movie *Midnight Express* very well; I was not about to get caught in another country breaking the law.

One of the highlights of being in Acapulco was the music performance I gave. I heard the band playing and I wanted to jam with those guys. I told one of my managers that I should sing with them and he told me to do it. Well, I went up and asked the band if they knew a few different songs and they said yes. I waited a minute and it was time to do my thing. I sang *Fresh* by Kool & the Gang, and ripped it! I sang in front of thousands of people from all over the world. It was a wonderful feeling being accepted and

appreciated by people from all over the world that evening.

One of the most exciting musical experiences was being in
the studio with Fred McFarlane. When I met him he was playing
keys for *James "D Train" Williams*. Fred and I learned that we
knew many of the same people in the business. He stayed busy. He
produced and wrote for Jenny Burton, Evelyn King, Intrigue, and I
think the Aleems. He really hit it big with Jocelyn Brown and
Somebody Else's Guy, I would go to the studio with him and his
music partner George Allen.

I was in the studio with Fred, George, and Jocelyn, as they
were working on her next follow up to *Somebody Else's Guy* and
in the studio next door was Diana Ross and Arthur Baker, the man
responsible for the early recordings of New Edition. I'll never
forget it because MTV was debuting Prince's song, *When Doves
Cry*. They blasted that joint in the studio. I thought I was going to
lose my mind. Diana Ross, Arthur Baker, Jocelyn Brown, Fred
McFarlane were so excited. I decided to leave; it was too much for
me. I kept saying to myself, leave so that you maintain some
control. Fred told me later that I should not have left. Diana Ross
came into the studio with them and everybody was jamming
together. I couldn't believe it.

Fred gave me a chance to do the response to Somebody
Else Guy, and I was sitting in his studio stuck on stupid. I couldn't
think of an idea, phrase, line or anything. I was so disappointed

and embarrassed at myself. So much experience and exposure through the years and here I was like a deer stuck in headlights. . A few weeks later, I started hearing this rap about *Somebody Else's Guy* with the same styled music. I really blew my shot.

One very good highlight was that Fred wrote a track for me called *Economy*; I was performing at a showcase down in midtown. Fred asked me if I was sure I wanted to sing about the economy and I was like, yep. So the day came for the show and there was a roster of talent. When Fred showed up, it was my turn to perform and I aced it. He thought that I had the best performance, but that damn concept of the *Economy*...the track didn't get promoted beyond that performance.

Another opportunity was presented when I began branching off from the band. I met one of the personnel from Ray, Goodman and Brown's entourage. They were looking for someone to open for their group and some new material. My contact's name was Fred. I gave him a tape, went down to the studio but my sound was not what they were looking for. Harry Ray went solo, and. Kevin Owens, who sang back up with Luther Vandross got the part.

Meanwhile, Louie moved to Rhode Island, I would eventually move to DC, and everybody just went into separate endeavors. We started talking about a reunion and got together, but it was not the same. Louie and I came up from DC, and Rhode Island, we went to the Bronx and met up with Ron, his lady,

James, and Dorian. It was good seeing everyone; it just didn't

turn out the way Ron was selling it.

We started playing some cover tunes first. Then I started to

notice that every time Louie and I would shout out to play one of

the originals, Ron would say something to divert the attempt. The

one original we played was *Black Rock* simply because the song

had the most basic chord structure of any classic rock song. I was

pretty pissed about that, and so was Lou. Then my homeboy had

the nerve to ask everybody to chip in towards some gas & electric,

man please.

I started recording with this cat named Julian Greene. Now,

I remember Julian was a few years younger than I was. I would see

him in the neighborhood when I first started singing with the choir

then later as I became a professional temp and got assignments on

Wall Street. We would do sessions in his home studio; right there

in the St. Nick projects. The sessions were tight and clean. We did

a bunch of songs that never went anywhere but still always

pressing towards the mark to make my name known. Julian had

about four acts; his old lady, a female rap group, a male rapper,

and me. We created press kits and I had to come up with a name.

Julian said "How about Sir Charles?" My response was, "Sure,

whatever!" The name stuck and I've been known as Sir Charles

ever since.

This was when Teddy Riley was hitting hard and *New Jack*

Swing was about to blow up. Right there in St. Nick projects on

127th Street I met Ted, and it was so funny; he was so shy and soft spoken. He was probably suspicious of everyone around him because Guy was blowing up, Johnny Kemp was just about to drop too and Keith Sweat was doing it big. By the way, I can't stand Keith. He had the nerve to tell me I couldn't sing. A few years prior to his major success, Keith was doing his thing with a group called Jamillah. They were opening for everybody, Teddy Pendergrass, and a bunch of folks. I think they played the Apollo, and that joint on 91st Street and Columbus Avenue. But this whinny-nosed, begging, singing Negro was so high on himself, I couldn't take it. Now besides his begging style, I do not have anything against the brother, but do not pull me down because you are about to blow up.

I stopped recording with Julian and started hanging with Greg Birch. Birch and I started recording in his crib using computers across from the projects on 127th Street. Now, through this entire time I had started using crack and wouldn't stop for a long time. Birch had a Juno keyboard, a Macintosh computer, and we had to write about a dozen songs. We were like Michael Franks and Mic Murphy from The System. We tried to get deals, but nothing would fall into place.

After Birch and I went our separate ways, I ran into Billy Jones, the former lead singer of The Moments of Truth. The group had an album and as a teenager, I remember catching one of their gigs on Lenox Avenue. Years later, when I ran into Billy, I was sure to let him know I remembered catching the show. It made him feel good that he was remembered and that he was appreciated.

Billy saw that I was hungry and a hustler, so we started talking about the possibility of getting something together. Billy kept saying we need lots and lots of practice, so we met in some of the community centers in St. Nick projects to rehearse. It was me and two other guys, but it was not meant to be and we just stopped meeting.

By then, I was working in midtown in the Garment District on 35th Street. I was right down the street from Macy's. I met my son's godfather by chance. I sold this dude a VCR tape of Muhammad Ali, and made that area my home base because the customers got to know me well and I made a lot of money. Ray and I made some contacts, and I started recording in the lower east side. John Roc and Eddie Matos were producing the music and musical arrangements while Ray and I would write lyrics, arrange vocals, and record them. We did at least a dozen songs, until Little Louie Vega asked for one of them on DAT. Then of course we never heard from him again and our song, *Something's Got To Give* was ghost.

A long time ago our choir director told us to stop trying to be stars because stardom is not meant for everyone. He said that sometimes we might have to settle for being a star in your own community, just in your own neighborhood. I didn't want to hear it but I knew it was true. Today I still sing produce music. I would love for God to bless my talents at least once on a national level, but if not I can't complain. I have done so much in this lifetime it's been amazing.

I have noticed in recent years that music has changed. I do not have an interest in it like I use to. Maybe I've lost some of my passion because I cannot hit the notes that I use to hit. I have to pick songs for performing very carefully. If you do not use it you will lose it. I lost a lot of my natural oomph. Now I work harder to get what I want musically. One of the most hurtful music experiences I had was when I was jamming with some cats that stayed on the road. I'll just call them "the road dogs." These guys played overseas, and when they came home they had fat pockets and performed all of the time. A few of the guys were thinking about getting their own group together because they had made so many connections and didn't want to be in the background.

At that time I use to gig in the subway after work with this girl named Alicia, and these other cats. We'd jam in the New York City Transit Authority subway all evening everyday if possible. We would make between fifty to one hundred dollars per night each. We would cover songs like Lou Rawls', *You'll Never Find*, Kool & the Gang's, *Too Hot*, old Motown, and all the good stuff. The New York tourists and white folks loved it. I would always rush home to get some crack and smoke my money up. The crack was calling me bad at that time.

It was a vicious cycle, always chasing the unobtainable.

The road dogs were backing up groups like Jeff Redd, Keith Sweat, and many of the artists that were hot when New Jack Swing was hitting. Here I am a bona fide singer and crack head jamming with them, but not hitting the mark because of my drug use. That was the only time I've been with a band and asked to leave. The group lost credibility because of me. Although, they had no proof about my lifestyle their assumptions were right. That hurt me to my core. I was in my late thirties and it was time to take notice of self. They were taking my mistress called music away from me.

Well anyway…the road dogs would rehearse once a week. This was around the time when "Remember The Time" was hitting hard! They had a connection that was going to get us some gigs, and the guys met one day and said they didn't think I fit the mode. When Al told me, I was crushed. The one thing that I had all of my life was not good enough. I know I was a pitiful drug addict, but not my music…I could still sing…couldn't I? My notes were flat, my wind was short, and I looked skinny and ashy. Deep down inside I knew it, I was just hoping for a pass. If I'd gotten the pass I would have messed up anyway. It was reality check time.

I may not have hit the big time, but I've done many things. Some big and some are just things that many people will never be able to do. I've been in so many studios, professional and otherwise. I've performed before thousands and met so many people in entertainment. When I think about Len Bias, that other cat that use to play for the Celtics, Rick James, David Ruffin, Eddie Kendricks, and Donny Hathaway I think about all of the drugs that I've done and I am still breathing. I've had a blessed life. If I were to die tomorrow I couldn't complain one bit. I thank God for all of my experiences. When I finally got clean I experienced for the first time how to perform without being high. I led a chorus at the substance abuse program, by singing in a twenty five hundred seat auditorium in Queens College. Oh yes, I was nervous and there were no drugs. I learned to feel that natural rush of adrenaline and I've been getting used to it for a while now. I've been clean now for over fifteen years and like the thirst for cool clean water, I want music that bad at times. I guess music was and still is one of my addictions.

Chapter 17

RELATIONSHIPS

We put ourselves in relationships that give us plenty of reason for pause. We do some of the same things over and over, substituting people and substituting places or things only to get the same results. I see why the old fashioned virtues lean towards not having serious involvement until you are certain of yourself and the person you are choosing to call your mate. I also understand the flip side of the coin, but it's not like tender feelings get tender mercy. It does not matter what type of person you are; if something happens to you, you just have to deal with it.

Now if you have God in your life you will be prepared for the ups and downs of life. I am sure your outlook will be different. I was trying to hold it all together when the family started to come together for a second or third time. Pete was moving in with us on Gerard Avenue in the Bronx. I wanted him to know that I could handle myself on the street and that I had connections. When he wanted herb I showed him who had what and where to go. He still relied on me to get it for him and truthfully, on the inside I wanted him to. I had continued my rise to the top of my bottom. I was on my way to King of the Woolahs. A woolah is a joint of cracked-laced reefer. I introduced Pete to crack cocaine. In some sick way I did what the streets expected me to do. Grab someone else and try to introduce him or her to all the negativity you can, but call it cool, and if you are lucky they will fall off, ruin their life, or die.

Is it a perfect life yet? We started smoking woolahs left and right. I was already smoking like crazy with my friends from the neighborhood. Tracy and I didn't really need any partners, but Pete was new to the neighborhood and I had to introduce him to the family that had adopted me. In return, he met others in the neighborhood that was from the old school too. I called them Harlem alumni. Pete was no leach. He paid his way and wanted to know what the next man was bringing to the table. This was good and bad. I soon adopted the same principle. I prevented people from leaching on to me, but I started to become very self-indulgent. It seems like I did drugs like people breathe air and after rolling at that pace for a while I found out Pete's heart couldn't take the processed cocaine. It was really messing him up. Meanwhile, I was smoking it like a kid eats candy. He had to leave it alone. In fact, he went back to snorting cocaine because it didn't have the same effect on his system. Most normal people with normal intelligence would say just leave it alone, but that is not the way of the streets. It is supposed to not make sense to make sense. Are you following me?

I moved in with Walter over on Macomb's Place, Skip, Walter's god-brother came out of nowhere and moved in also. We called each other brothers. Once again I was adopted into a family that cared about me and me about them. Skip had court cases and at the time we didn't know how things would play out for him. Walter's apartment was on the fourth floor and I finally snagged an apartment on the fifth floor when one became available. I'll never forget it; we had the craziest birthday party. My birthday was in November and Walter and Skips birthdays were in December, it was the bomb. We had two apartments filled with music. There were people in the hallways, on the staircases, and in both apartments; talk about off the hook. There were so many people there that I would meet people and take them to the fourth or fifth floor and then I'd forget that they were there. Those were some pretty wild times. I eventually lost my apartment and a lot of personal belongings. Why? Why else, because of drugs again. I was getting credit from a pretty decent guy from El Salvador, and I took advantage of myself and refused to pay bills.

In between relationships with Kim and Sunny I started playing the field off and on. I started seeing a young lady by the name of Charlene. She was nice. Real nice on the bottom, small on the top and she had a cute personality. We worked at the same bank. After Sunny was out of the picture, I started seeing Charlene exclusively. . I knew she was interested because her eyes told me so. I found out that she had been dating this guy named Charles. One day, he told her he didn't want to deal with her anymore and she almost had a nervous breakdown behind it because they were living together.

When Charlene and I met she wanted to know up front what my intentions were. I told her that I liked her and I was not seeing any one. Of course I wanted to get with her, but I never had the skills to get with a woman without assuring her I was not running game on her. It seemed that I always had to commit. I was not sure how to talk to women at times. I was never the rapper or the Don Juan type. Strangely enough, since Charlene was just getting over a situation with a guy she would eventually play me the same way he played her years later.

We started this relationship on sort of false pretenses. I found out her loss caused her to have a need for someone and I seemed to have a need for a lover. I really was not ready for a descent relationship at the time. I was still numb from breaking up with Sunny. Charlene was a very charming girl and very sincere. Our relationship began to flourish. We went to parties together and hung out a lot. By the time I moved to Macomb's we seemed to adjust to one another fairly well. My mother liked Charlene a lot too.

They would go shopping together and talk with one another very often. My mother seemed to be trying to give Pete another chance. He'd left his place in Harlem and moved in with my mom and sister Monique. At that time had adjusted to the neighborhood. I lost my apartment and moved back with the family on Gerard Avenue. The family was looking into the possibility of moving back to Manhattan. My Aunt Marie was very sick at that time. My mother would try and spend as much time with her as possible in her last days. My Aunt was very instrumental in arranging an apartment in her building. The family took the apartment and soon after my aunt passed on. We took over her apartment, so there was a double move. Charlene and I continued to see one another. I left the apartment with my family and moved into Pete's apartment on 127th Street.

The reason I do not believe in coincidence is simply because of how my life has unfolded. Now when you read about me talking about God and it seems that I am changing the flavor or direction of the book honestly, I am not. How can I explain almost falling off a cliff numerous times and in numerous situations? I can't explain it. There has to be an explanation or divine intervention. Just like the Jenkins family in Manhattan when I was approaching adulthood or the Hayes family during my college years or even the Brown family after the college years. The relationships I've had with these families that seem to adopt me were peculiar.

I think it was God's way of holding on to me protecting me for later in life. It's not like I never got hurt physically or mentally, but it could have been so much worse. Suppose they were never there. There is no telling what my life would have been like. It seemed as if they viewed me as a white collar, educated type of brother from around the way that was down to earth, but had a little dirt under his nails. Now on the other hand, they worked odd jobs, in some cases they hustled and I knew that, it has been part of my life all my life at one point or another. The main difference seemed to be cash flow.

When you hang out with people that do not work consistently you have to be careful of expectations and you need to know boundaries. You have to be able to hold your own. I am no sucker, but if we are hanging with each other then we need to be contributing together. When it comes to buying a bottle, a bag, or going to the movies I am not pimping anybody and nobody is pimping me. I found out the hard way that close friends and family will play you unless you make it clear where you are coming from. I was and still feel very close to all of the families. I have not seen some of them in years and it would not matter, because I still have love for them.

Having no money can be overlooked depending on what else one brings to the table. Now that isn't saying a lot if one person spends a lot of money every day, but there is more to relationships than money. There are times when life is like a seesaw. Things that are important can have a varying effect on us at various times depending on what's happening in our lives at that moment. If I needed somebody to have my back Tracy would be there, if I wanted or needed a partner to roll with Tracy was there, Carlton would be there too. If girls were involved they both were there. Pete and I wound up getting credit from an old timer in the area named Louie. We could get whatever we wanted, crack or cocaine. I mismanaged money very badly back in the day. I took money from my job and put it back. I would borrow money from my mother. I even worked the streets at lame odds and ends jobs, as well as sold some of my personal belongings. I did

everything that I could to keep up a healthy drug habit.

Fred had a Tom's route. Tom's is the East Coast candy

company that distributes chips, cupcakes, and snacks. Fred was

pretty successful and was looking for someone to tutor, franchise,

his efforts. He used to have seizures and it was time for him to

slow down. Fred lived in the building on the corner of 157th

between Walton Avenue and Gerard Avenue. He was really a good

guy. He bought a store in the neighborhood and used his franchise

to fill it. He helped Tracy get a licensed gun and began preparing

him to take over his route. He gravitated to Tracy and me because

he knew I worked for a living and Tracy was respected in the

neighborhood.

Fellas see you coming and they want that energy that you

have. You have to preserve all that you have for yourself and your

success. Fred's health was failing him and he died. I worked two

jobs (I was a bank teller a local commercial bank and a parking

attendant at Kinney's Garage); I performed with a band. I guess I

was supposed to have money. As people gravitated to me, I

allowed it. I started messing around eventually because Kim and I

would have vicious arguments. Things changed drastically. Kim

accused me of fooling around, which was not true, yet. She took

the baby and moved in with her mother on Webster Avenue. Kim

was a very interesting and attractive girl, but her sexual experience

was limited. I was not interested in teaching just appreciating. I know sometimes you have to teach or tell a person what you want in order to get it, but I was not going there. I wanted whomever I dealt with to be just as versatile or open as I was. It may be unfair, but these are some of the things we learn in life.

One thing about my drug life, I didn't know God was with me all the time. I was just too high to know it then. God gives us freedom of choice and I wanted to belong so bad that I abused my freedom of choice until it became slavery. I became a slave to all of the drugs in my life and fell in love with the lifestyle. In previous chapters I mentioned the quiet voice that would tell me not to get high, or the voice would say "You are not supposed to do that." The more I got high the quieter the voice became. I lied to myself for a very long time and I actually tried to convince myself that I had everything under control.

I tried to murder my conscious spirit by pouring more and more substance into my body. As years passed by I heard the innocent voice less and less. Let me show you how good God has been. He allowed me to fall deeper in debt and despair so that he could be the one to rescue me. Being arrested, using drugs was not a lifestyle for me, but God knew that if I was left to my own devices I would mess up. Hopefully, because the ground work or the foundation of a Christian life was taught to me as a child, I would have something to fall back on, I would have someone to cry out to, someone to hear my plea and he heard me, and saved me. He saved me through my guilt. He saved me through the eyes of my children. He simply gave me an opportunity to have a second lease on life. I would have to recognize him for God and I would realize he was in charge.

Had it not been for the fact I am from a loving family that raised me on a Christian belief system I would have never been where I am today. I would not have had the opportunity to work in one of the most important government agencies in the world. It is an agency that has shown me trust, and they desire to invest money into me for specialized training. They are allowing me, a drug addict to teach other people how to speak, conduct themselves, and how to use customer service skills. Imagine that a drug addict for over twenty-five years is now positioned to teach people about things that I was not able to be taught until later in my life.

God was there. It's not a perfect life but it is my life. There are people in this world that have never used drugs a day in their lives and they have not had the opportunities that I have had. I have survived being arrested, being incarcerated, being a drug addict, just living and breathing in the bowels of ghetto life, but I only made it by the grace of God.

I was down in the muck and filth of life with no one and nothing to call my own. I didn't have much of anything, just a little bit of love. My life was screaming to be heard, seen, and held. It was screaming because of the unknown and desperately wanting to be significant. The previous pages and chapters should have told you where I was, it was not a good place. I am not the same person—that drug addict, manipulator, and self-centered

person—just looking for his next high. I didn't care if it was drugs, sex or an opportunity to make some fast cash. Today I live for Christ and I am still growing, and learning. I am still trying, I am still being challenged and tested and I thank God for it. I told someone recently that when people say you are a trip, it is better to be a trip than the destination. When you are all about the trip there is so much to see, learn, experience, test, taste, and observe. But, if you are about the destination, it's all over. My heart and soul was convicted because of how I was living.

The way I was living was not right. I was not being the right example for my children; I was not being the right example for my spouse, more importantly I was not being the right example for a child of God. Sure, I had my moments, we all do. But the overall picture was not good. The Lord challenged me, he made me look at myself and the guilt was too great. I couldn't bear the burden. I had to face myself for who I was, and I was nobody taking up space in a body once owned by a child of God. My dad told me a long time ago that if you can't look at yourself in the mirror, you have got a problem. I didn't understand that statement as an eleven-year-old boy, but as a man of thirty-four years of age I couldn't stare in the mirror at myself. Those words came back to me ringing in my head.

My face was gaunt, my teeth were stained from smoking cigarettes, marijuana and cocaine, my breath smelled even when I would brush them, my eyes were sunken in and usually blood shot, my hair was un-kept and I sweated profusely, my clothes were always baggy or too big. I couldn't stand the sight of that person anymore. The Lord had convicted me through the eyes of my children just in case I had reservations. But today I claim the victory. I can't say that I have a perfect life, but I keep striving towards the mark. If I can do what I have done, there is no doubt in my mind that you can also. I no longer have guilt, or shame, because I can do all things through Christ that strengthens me.

Surrendering from drugs was such a huge ordeal, and I mean huge with a capital HUGE! The day I went to Harlem Hospital to surrender the psychiatrist they made interview me told me that I was very smart and that my insight could prove beneficial if I was not an addict. I am not claiming brilliance, but I think that sort of stayed in the back of my mind somewhere. After his series of questions, he asked me if I would take a bed if one became available to me.

I agreed immediately, not knowing what was in store for me. Somehow I managed to have about forty dollars left in my pocket. My appointment at Harlem Hospital's psych ward was at ten o'clock in the morning. I remember feeling like I was about to receive a new lease on life. I went home, bought a stem and about thirty dollars' worth of crack and began the journey to a new chapter in my life. I stayed up all night trying to re-smoke what was already gone.

Trueality Enterprises

The next day I made it to my appointment and sat around for what seemed to be an eternity. I watched the clock, doctors, and nurses only to watch the clock some more. Then finally, we were off to get a bed and start the recovery process. Harlem Hospital is on 135th Street and Lenox Avenue, but it actually takes up the entire square block. They had found a location off site, no more than ten minutes away. When we got there they showed us where we were supposed to bunk and get settled. As we began to look around we found out that there was a psych ward right there, but it was fenced off.

Nobody was permitted in the psych ward without an escort because these patients had serious and severe mental health problems. I was there because I was a drug addict and I kept saying to myself, "I am not crazy, why they had to send me here?" Meanwhile, there were patients already at the facility when we arrived. I made the assumption that they had drug problems. I was right, but there was more. They were patients with drug problems and mental instability issues too.

We needed to be there for ten days until we could get to the facility that would actually house us. I couldn't wait to get out of the psych ward. I literally counted the days, and it took forever. I made friends with one guy that seemed quite normal, but he got a kick out of pissing off one of the psych patients. The guy he upset was about six-foot-four and he weighed about three hundred pounds. Big-man just pointed, saying, "I am going to get you!" I was so emotionally shattered, not to mention skinny there was

nothing I could do. The showdown would be the next day and I

was not sure how it would play out however, it started just like all

of the others.

We would get our routine going by getting up and doing

the things which should have been normal like washing, making up

your bed, etc. but for an addict, it was not the first train of thought.

We were taking babies steps in getting our lives back on track. Just

before lunch Big-man came out into the dayroom and pointed to

me saying, "I know you had nothing to do with it, but your friend

is going to get it." I really do not know what my friend did to upset

this dude, but I knew it was not me and I would not have been

trying to piss anybody off. For me, being in treatment was all about

trying to get my life together. I didn't feel like it, but my soul was

dying. Scamming people or trying to pull the wool over someone's

eyes is one thing when you are on drugs and they are not. Things

escalate to another level when you talk about interacting with

someone that has psychological problems compounded with

chronic drug use.

I would eventually end up at a facility known as Samaritan

Village. The first Samaritan Village stop was in Queens, NY.

That's where I traded my drug habit for an official cigarette habit.

They gave us cigarettes on a regular basis. In the long run it would

be another hard habit to break. They had facilities all over the city.

I was moved to the Bronx from Queens, and that is where I stayed to finish my treatment. The hurting thing was, at that location I could see the neighborhood that I did all of my drugging in. For a while it was like torture, seeing the neighborhood and knowing that my children were there but I couldn't see them. Actually, I could have walked out at any time and left but I was committed to the process, and I was afraid for my life. There were three programs at Samaritan Village, an A, B, and C plan.

I believe the A plan was for your typical addict with all of the encounter groups and education courses built in. That is just the way they did it at that time. The B plan was for mandated patients that had a criminal record, repeat offenders that used drugs, and a last time opportunity to prevent them from going to jail by basically blaming your problem on drug use. Then the C plan was a new program that had already run its course by the time I had arrived. The group of people that came in with me would be the last to be enrolled under that classification. Who in the world can use drugs for ten, twenty or more years and just stop in six months? Anything is possible, but I started to wonder if they ever expected it to be a success. When you think about the conspiracy theories, you have to think about practical situations that you can identify with personally.

For example, Cancer has been running rampant in our country for years. Why have they not found a cure or gotten closer to one? With all of the drugs that people use how do they get into the United States? Who allows or prevents it? Who benefits when people get caught distributing or selling drugs? Who benefits when people do not get caught? It is a vicious cycle and you do not need a degree to know that. Did they give us cigarettes to rid the world of us via Cancer? Did they create a six-month program knowing most would not be successful and when we failed they could officially lock us up?

It was a good opportunity for me because then I could get my life back. I could have my children back in my life, and hopefully now that I had that, I have an opportunity to give back to the world and capture that elusive significance that I once mentioned. I started to wonder about the truth in all of the things that I learned and was exposed to. I do not know what you believe, but I know from what I've gone through there has to be a God and not just any God. I believe in Jesus Christ. I do not believe he had blonde hair and blue eyes, but if Christ word stands as truth and he died for all people, it really should not matter what color his eyes, skin, or hair were.

He saved me when nobody else would or could. I have practiced Buddhism and Islam, yet to me Christianity is where I belong. I have mad respect for other cultures and religions. The extremist are another story. The Torah, The Quran, The Book of Life, nor The Bible promotes violence and senseless killing. I know that God is OMNI-PRESENT and ONIPOTENT. I still make mistakes in fact I probably make mistakes daily, but God is a merciful God and he allows me the opportunity to grow and learn.

For that alone, I praise him.

My desire to be a Public Speaker is to share the good news.
I do not want to beat people down with the Bible or biblical
principles, but would like to let them know from whence have
come. I would like to let those that are down, lost, or unsure know
that life can be good, and if it is already good it can be great. If you
do not have a perfect life, it is ok, just strive for a pure heart. God
bless you all.

Chapter 18

DIVORCE

In this book I talk a lot about relationships, learning about women, and engaging them intimately. There have been a lot of lessons learned and none mastered. Dealing with the opposite sex is an ongoing life lesson. I know a lot, but not nearly enough. Maybe it is just that I refuse to play the game that society has laid out for centuries, I imagine. You know the dance. Some of it is ok, but I just can't get with a lot of the relationship stereotypes. The stereotypes that relate to some of the courting process, you know the old cat and mouse game. The fact of the matter is men and women want the same things in life primarily, but we are supposed to play the lady and gentleman role, so that it measures out properly in the eyes of our society. Ok, call me a caveman.

Then there is the baby momma drama and child support stereotypes that are just sickening. You know the scenarios. "Get that money girl." That is crazy, that women live with and off of the set up and exploitation of this mindset. There are times when it is appropriate, but it just seems to be so relevant in the minds of women. Especially the way things are accentuated and portrayed in movies, videos, and reality shows.

The blessings in my life are many yet they sometimes seem few. My wife came into my life at a time when I started to take life serious. We met a year or two before I got clean. We met in a bus terminal in Washington, D.C. on our way back to New York. Now that seems like something you would read in a book or see in a movie.

The truth of the matter it was an innocent interaction between two people with no strings attached, that is until a conversation started. I saw her in the bus terminal and she struck me before I even saw her face. It was the black. Black is my favorite color and she had on black from head to toe. Long flowing braids, a long black leather coat, black boots and I took notice immediately. At that time, I was still using drugs heavily. I wanted to speak to her because I was attracted right away. I made up my mind in the very next instant that I would not say anything because I couldn't go anywhere with it. Why waste time trying to talk to a woman when you are already in a relationship, and that relationship is on the rocks.

I am addicted to drugs; and my relationship is in the toilet with the mother of my two children. Just as all of that became glaringly obvious the intrigue died. I asked her if I was at the bus gate for the departure to New York, she confirmed that I was in the right place. Nothing more was said between us at the time, my initial interest was still slowly fading away. I looked around to see what time it was or where the rest of the people were because going to New York from anywhere is generally crowded. I turned back around and she had disappeared. The bus pulled up, I got on and a few seconds later I look up and she is saying "I think I know you from somewhere". I couldn't believe it. I started saying to myself, here we go, that is supposed to be the guys line? Here it is I am trying to mind my business and do the right thing and she is talking about knowing me.

She inquired about my job and activities. I thought it was possible she could have seen me on television, because I've sung around town and have done a lot of music things in my life. Nope, that was not it. It turns out she knew me from the old neighborhood in Harlem. Actually our families knew each other. We talked on the bus all the way to New York. When it was all said and done we exchanged numbers. My interest was definitely piqued again! I just didn't know what would come out of it. We left each other with a peck on the cheek.

I called her a couple of weeks later and was supposed to meet her. Little did I know, she was telling everyone that she had met her future husband, and I was still torn between scratching up money to go meet her and scratching up the money to get high. I didn't know whether I could make up a good excuse to get away from the house and the kids to go see a woman that wanted to be with me. I stood her up twice. I was so embarrassed I didn't even bother to call her again. Let's face it, when you meet someone that is attractive and you both seem to like each other, then you decide to hook up but don't, what is the likelihood of there being any further interest. I chalked it up as water under the bridge.

I had a life altering experience. I couldn't stand my drug use anymore. I couldn't look at myself in the mirror. My heart was broken every time I looked at my children. I had hit bottom and I didn't know what to do about it. The one thing I knew was that something had to change, and it was me! I couldn't enjoy the drugs and I didn't enjoy my life anymore. I went into a drug program. My girl and I were both supposed to go, but she reneged. She may have had one or two sessions with a counselor, but when I committed myself, she used that as an opportunity to move to New Jersey with her sisters and in-laws. I went anyway. I held a strong resentment towards her for her trickery or whatever, but it is behind me now.

Halfway through the program I had a conversation with one of my fellow inmates in the program. He asked me why I didn't have any visitors. I told him of my baby momma drama and that all of my support was coming from my family that was out of town. In fact, my mom and my sister Cecelia came from D.C. to the Bronx to visit me with a crazy care package. They bought underwear, long johns, shirts, pants, a coat and the whole nine . I was blown away by the love. I knew they loved me, but I just didn't see it coming. I guess I should have expected it. The moment I left home and started falling off the path of how I was raised, they would call me to encourage me, or send me cards, or letters to make sure that I remembered how I was reared.

Then I remembered that I had Renee's number he pushed me to call her. I was afraid because I left her hanging not once but twice. I took the chance and called Renee. She was surprised and happy to hear from me. That call meant a lot to me also. We

began writing each other, and I started calling her on the regular.

My kids would eventually come to visit me although their mom

had made up her mind she and I was over. I was still grateful to

have some time with Charles and Sasha. I love those kids so much.

My daughter Kychel didn't come to see me. I was so emotionally

tapped; maybe I never told her mother where I was. Like I said, it

took some time, but I got over the deception.

Renee would eventually come to visit me. And when I was

given a weekend pass which enabled me the opportunity to go out

on a visit without supervision, she was the first person that I went

to visit. I was upfront with Renee the entire time she and I were in

communication. I told her about my progress, my status, my

intentions, and everything. After all, I was trying to lead my life in

a different direction. It was a special time in my life. Most

importantly I was able to share that time with Renee. I really

wanted everything in order. Not only did I go into the program but

I completed the program including aftercare and graduation.

The big deal with completing a drug program is that most

addicts do not complete anything in their lives. I do not have the

exact numbers, but I am pretty sure the ratio or percentages are low

for those that complete and do not go back to using again. As

Renee and I got closer and closer I thought our relationship should

be on a different level. I lived in the Bronx and she lived in Long

Island with her kids.

In hindsight I now know we should have taken more time to get to know each other, but things are usually going to happen in one way or another and for her and I they happened pretty quickly. After dating for a few months, we decided that we were going to be married and that is exactly what we did. My mother told me not to do it, and the program advised against serious decisions before one year of completing the program. The only upsetting thing for me is that my children were not in the wedding.

The judge ordered their mom to make sure that they would be included, and she mucked it up. She was scared of repercussion, because I was not playing games with her at this point. I was telling the judge any and everything that I thought was foul. Raw feelings and new attitude can make you go there. The wedding was a success regardless. I use to say that when I got married it would be like the movie *Bachelor Party* with Tom Hanks. I wanted chicks and guns and fire engines "Whoo-hoo!" Now that was true when I was getting high and doing drugs but after I got clean, I didn't care about those things. I didn't even want a bachelor party. One of the most exciting things to happen was at my reception. We had a DJ, and people from both sides of the family were there. Her side of the family was down to Earth regular folk. That is something you just have to be able to appreciate. My family was from the traditional church side of the tracks.

I sang at my wedding and it was well received by my
wife and all of our friends and family in attendance. From that
point forward it was a different kind of work that I was not used to.
The first couple of years I couldn't believe that I was married, but
the feeling passed and I recognize that it was what it was.

My wife and I had some rocky times. We struggled and
fought hard with and for our relationship, but I felt in my heart that
she loved me and really meant well. That is one of the most
important things in a relationship. Although the marriage was a
blessing, some things do not always turn out the way you intend or
want them to. It is sad to say that, since the original writing of this
passage we have divorced.

If you asked me, I would say the failure of the divorce fell
on the shoulders of both of us, but in different areas. Sometimes
the psychological effects of a relationship may be just as hard to
see, to accept, or to understand. I can admit and accept the role I
played in the failure of the relationship. I can only imagine that she
does also. In the end I chose to initiate the steps to end our nine-
year marriage. When it was all said and done it was about ten years
and some change. I hate the fact that I failed at something as
serious as marriage, and I failed vows promised before God. We
were at a point that there were so many arguments and really bad
ones at times. We both agreed to separate if things didn't get
better, and they didn't get better. I started the process of looking
for a place to go and did just that. After we both moved, we would

try to be normal but it seemed to be too odd. After a final argument we stopped seeing each other. There was no warning or discussion about it we just stopped calling and dating.

I think men are usually a bit cold and non-caring when it comes to a relationship being over. I began to become numb to the idea of not seeing her, but we were still legally married. Life goes on, so I started the process of getting the divorce proceedings together. Building up to the finale, was draining. I didn't realize how much we still were attached emotionally. It can be that you still love or are in love with the person that you married or it could simply be that although you are going in separate directions at that point you still acknowledge what the relationship was supposed to be. Think about a tree that comes out the Earth and grows branches after a long time. It is the same tree but it has separate branches and they may not even face each other anymore, yet they are still from or part of the same tree. They start as one out of the Earth and begin leaning in different directions sometimes one side may get more sunlight than the other and the leaves seems more plentiful than other branches, but yet they are still a part of the same tree.

Getting a witness to swear before the courts, and having a relationship severed from a legal standpoint is no joke. After going back and forth to court there was one final appearance, and we would see each other for the l time. For me to see how visibly shaken and upset she was after all of this hurt me to my core. I thought about all that we went through in flashes and felt horrible.

I thought about how angry I was at times and all of the things that I did to contribute to our split, but I still had to do it for my sanity. A zebra won't change its stripes and neither does a leopard change its spots. If you think of it, it is just a shame that human beings can't or do not come clean with each other enough to make a relationship work. It is so much more than words and it is so much deeper too.

The healing process does not have a time frame on it. It too is what it is and can damage us for the rest of our lives. The truth of the matter is that this motivational speaker and child of God was just as taxed about the divorce as she was. It didn't matter that I initiated the process. There are times when you have to do what you need to do and that may cause you pain. It takes a lot of courage to face this type of decision and I do not look to putting myself in that position again at least no time soon anyway.

After a year or so I felt compelled to call and clear the air or give her a chance to give me a piece of her mind. I didn't want the latter, but I owed it to her because when she asked me to talk to her before the divorce, I couldn't do it. I was too emotional, the pain ran too deep, and once again it didn't matter that I was initiating the process. So I called her and she was ok with meeting to discuss whatever. I thought we both needed to address some closure issues that were never resolved. I never hated her, but I know that a man and a woman have a role in every relationship and the only time that changes is when that man and woman decide that they want their respective roles to be different. If that understanding is not held up, honored, or accepted, there is a void and a violation of that relationship. I am traditional but I am also straight up. When we met I did more talking than she did. It was important to make amends if possible. I am a lot to deal with, but I am not unfair or unreasonable unless someone is bringing that type of energy to me.

I've gone through traumatic changes in my life and probably have not taken adequate time to adjust in many situations. However, once I have decided to move forward I move forward. Trust me, it may not be in my best interest all of the time, but I am not taking no mess from anybody, and I am not trying to treat anyone with disrespect either.

Chapter 19

MILESTONES

It seems wild that I would be at a point in my life that I would write a book and consider the fact that I have milestones to talk about. Nevertheless, I do. The first thing of significance that comes to mind is the fact that completing something is the biggest difference maker of all. I finished high school, which generally speaking was easy, I didn't think so at the time but as I take everything into consideration it was.

Getting off drugs, now there's a milestone. Getting off and staying off is an accomplishment that most obsessives can't claim. It took me one and a half tries, but dag on it I have done it and I am grateful. I never thought after all of the years of abuse that I would be a complete person. I have my children back in my life, which to me is the most important thing in this world.

I have people who look at me with trust and respect as an individual and as a recovering addict. That is a bonus! I have a job that I have held down for over ten years and I am active in my community, I vote, and I am a game entrepreneur! My first tangible milestone was probably a CD titled *Cary's Standards*. I recorded three songs; *Misty, It Had to Be You, and All of Me*. I won second place in a local recording studio contest and won some studio hours as a result, and that afforded me the opportunity to add a fourth song. *Kissing A Fool by* George Michael to the standard CD. It was my first Executive Produced music project. I stayed on the local jazz circuit for a minute, mainly because I had a CD and it sounded pretty good. But, my main music preference was usually rhythm and blues with other musical influences laced in and around it.

I wrote my first book *Poetic Xpressions* around 2005, and started a poetry night in sunny downtown Suitland, Maryland at Cranberries. The Christmas CD, *Cary's Holiday* that was a free thank you to the community for all of the local support I was getting. There were many of the favorites like *The Christmas Song, White Christmas and What A Wonderful World.* I thought it was a nice touch during the Holiday season.

Due to the fact that I had been off of drugs for a few years at that time, I had begun speaking quite a bit and trying to find my niche. As a member of Toastmasters, I would climb through the ranks and become an Advance Toastmaster's Bronze, Competent Leader, and club Secretary, and club President. The very next logical step was to join the National Speaker's Association; I was so excited once I was accepted. I went to a convention in California and also joined the local chapter here in D.C.

I received the Director's Award of Excellence during 2007 for work I did during 2006 and 2007. I traveled around to different parts of the country on behalf of the Federal Reserve Law Enforcement Unit. My topics were primarily Customer Service or Public Speaking. I went to the Federal Reserves of Chicago,

Boston, Atlanta, and Detroit to facilitate classes on

professionalism. At the Board of Governors in Washington, D.C., I would usually teach classes annually. That is huge in my eyes. Not very often can a black man that used drugs get his life together. Let alone put together a lesson plan, be given a credit card with a few thousand dollars on it, and be trusted to travel around the country unsupervised while teaching and speaking/ On top of all of this I am rewarded at the end with a cash bonus and the acknowledgement of my peers. That is far from the norm at least when you come from where I am from.

From there I did some local gigging in the DMV. I decided to record audio to my book, *Poetic Xpressions*, because in my heart I thought it was a bit lack luster. I moved on to do several videos on *Fear, What's Your B Plan* and some other motivational topics. Eventually, I had to get back to music. I recorded a 17 track CD. It was a combination of which I executive produced, but I worked with various local producers, writers, vocalist, and DMV radio personalities. The title of the CD is Around the Mic with Sir Charles & Friends. That CD was debuted at an event called The Three Spokesmen If you do not know (DMV) stands for DC, MD, and VA.

A friend asked me if I was interested in auditioning for a movie. By chance, I landed a bit part in the movie *National Treasure-Book of Secrets*. That was a great experience working with Nicholas Cage, Ed Harris, Bruce Greenberg and Jon Voigt.

There are pictures of some of these activities in the book. As you may be able to tell, I have always stayed active. From there, I went on to start another weekly event Wordplay Wednesday, which was held at a Starbucks in Forestville, MD. The goal here was to provide a platform for artists to express their talent for free in the middle of the week. We had many, and some were the best. Sylvia Traymore Morrison, Ty Gray-El, Terrance the Comedian, She 7, Jus Me, Lamont Carey, Enoch the 7th Prophet, The Amazing Gospel Souls, Mahoganee, WOW Radio, Can We Talk Radio, and the list goes on, and on.

That event spawned the idea to have an informational community wide event. So I did it, under the name Help Us Help You. I had sponsors from all over the community like Giant, Verizon, Browns Market, Jerry's Subs & Pizza, PNC Bank, Starbucks, I mean we were running with some heavy hitters and it was all for the community. One good thing about milestones is that it is a way of measuring time, and what you have done in your life. Hopefully, when you reflect on the milestones of your life you are able to relish in the fact that you have done something that matters. That brings me to my alma mater, Norman Thomas High School. I found out the school was closing because of numbers. There are not as many graduates in schools across the country as there once were.

Our Norman Thomas HS graduating class of 1978 is second to none. I never realized the value and quality of the relationships that would be formed. There is a healthy majority of us that have tightly interwoven relationships and it is special. Mike Barlow, Veronica Frazier, Wayne Thomas, Sadler, Billy Taylor, Alicia Smith, Geoff Hinds, Jeff Anderson, Adrienne White, Janna Green, Renee Wilson, and so many others that have already been mentioned in previous chapters. To those that have not been mentioned, you are no less than the rest, but I've got to finish the story.

Brenda McLaughlin has been the matriarch of everything happening with everybody for the past thirty plus years so when I found out about the school closing I couldn't believe it. I spoke with the school liaison Debra Knight, who is also an alumni and she set it up for me to be the keynote speaker for the graduation ceremony. The class of 2009 would be mine to send out into the world, and they couldn't wait. Not to hear me, but to get out into the world. It was sad because our young have changed so much, but I was grateful to be able to give back to a school and a memory that meant so much to me as I grew up.

The very next milestone came to me unintentionally, as most probably do. I reluctantly responded to a casting call on *Facebook* to play an older character in a stage play. My girl Sharon told me that I should go for it, and I was feeling like whatever. I knew I could do it, but it was just about getting the details and committing to the part and the project. I knew the producer, Dawayne Williams and read for the part. They accepted me. It was a small part and I was ok with that, because I always have so much going on. I didn't want to commit to a part with a lot of lines.

I played his father, and finally got my part down and was ready to do the play. The play was performed at Suitland High School in Suitland, MD. We began with the opening act. I had quite a bit of time before my part and decided to record snippets in between scenes. I thought it would be pretty cool to have some footage. After the production was over, I put it together, and launched it to YouTube, and on Dawayne's Facebook page.

The play was titled after the book of the same name, Reputations Fade Away. It seems that a few folks saw it and liked it and he did too, apparently. And thus began the discussion, can you shoot a movie? We went on to shoot the film after several months and several scenarios and voila, another milestone! I shot my first full-length film. I had shot documentaries and music videos, but it added to my expertise as a filmmaker and it was a great opportunity to take all that I knew and use it for this project.

As I was wrapping up the shooting phase of the movie, I began getting sick. I had no idea what was really wrong with me so the decision had also been made to do a CD. I thought that maybe I should record my last recording as an artist, because I didn't have the time to do a lot of singing and performing. I found that I actually did a lot of videography. Either as documentary for

Sharon, myself as a speaker, or the potential to contract my services out became more and more lucrative.

As it turned out I had a couple of people that were interested in music for projects and most of my video work needed music. Why should I use someone else's music when I could create my own? The next milestones would be in creating my own music publishing company (SCC Music Production & Leasing) and an advertising production company (Affordable Advertising).

No matter how I twisted it, it was all me, Trueality Enterprises. It has kept me going and people are recognizing the brand. One way to look at milestones is very similar to how people see success, it is not always about dollars and cents, but it can be. I am very passionate about the things described in this book and I can do most of them for hours or even days without becoming bored. I love it and I am grateful for it, because I can continue to learn because of it!

MILESTONES

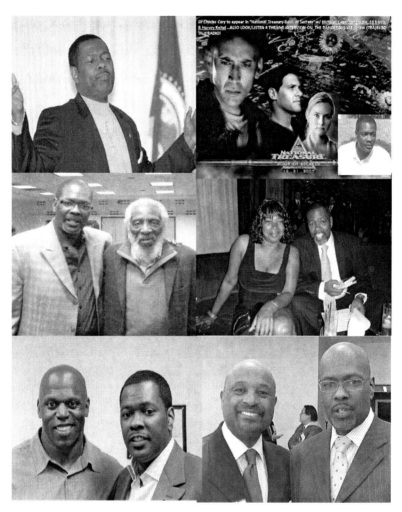

Performing at the Federal Reserve on occasion was great, meeting Dick Gregory at Howard University, Redskins great Ken Harvey, my bit part in National Treasure (Book of Secrets), My sweetie Sharon Parker of ROASA, & my main man Willie Jolley.

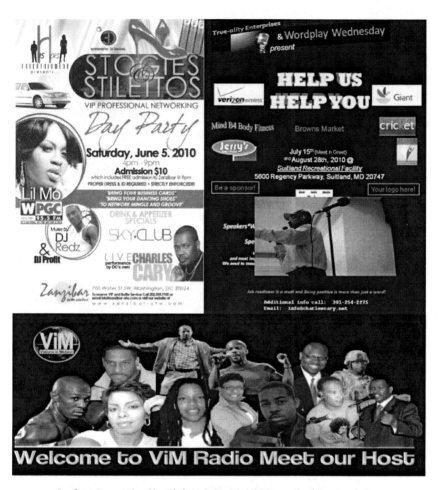

Performing at the Sky Club in DC with Lil Mo as the host, and the community event I put on (HELP US HELP YOU) was great. It's about giving back with sponsor support. I always had a blast with the VIM Radio network (Ted Harge, J'Ril, Mike the Solution Lee, Mari Torres, Dawn Mangham, Anita Charlot, Tim Miller, Jay King and gang) ...really great times.

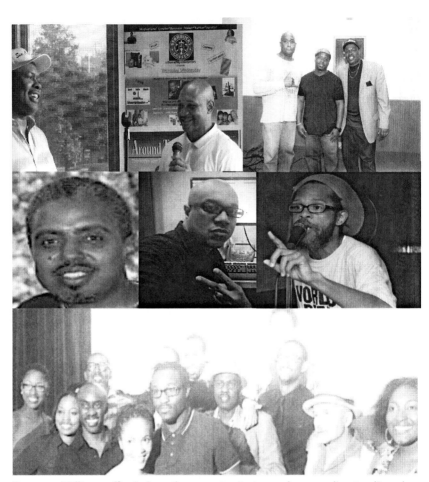

Dawayne Williams afforded me the opportunity to produce, co-direct, edit and score his movie Reputations Fade Away, Poety Man & David the Uncrowned King joined me for the "3 Spokesmen" Spoken-word performance, Kwan Taylor of "Skye Media" and Enoch of "El-Shamesh Photography" are great to work with. I learned so much from my friend Paul Laurence formerly of Hush productions...he's still making hits in my mind. Langston & Selton Shaw gave me a shot in their film "Dream Cash" with some all star actors.

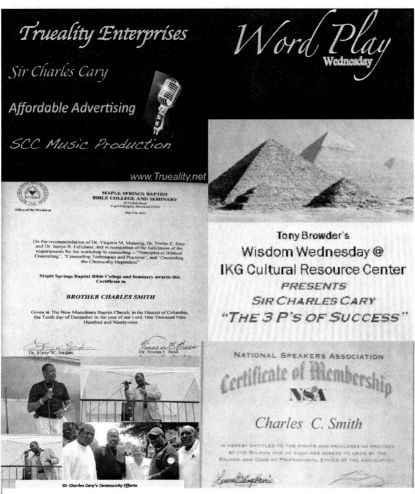

Wordplay Wednesday my weekly platform for artist of all types, Affordable Advertising gives me the opportunity create commercials Or promos for new, small, & indie's. Speaking at Tony Browders IKG Cultural Ctr gave me lots of exposure. Becoming certified counselor and a member of the National Speakers Association was glorious.

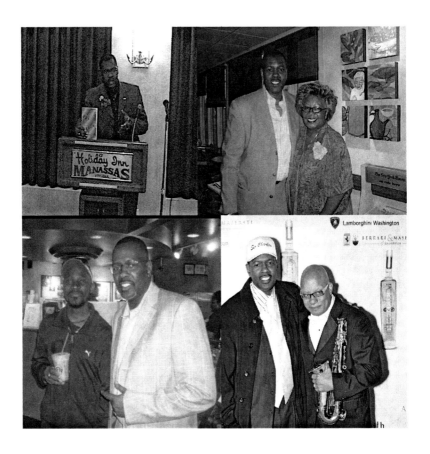

Speaking at the National Conference of Negro Women.
My publicist Reba Barnes.
Starbucks Mgr. John McKenna who is responsible for Wordplay
Wednesday.
Red Carpet Event w/Ski Johnson, Grammy Nominated Sax man.

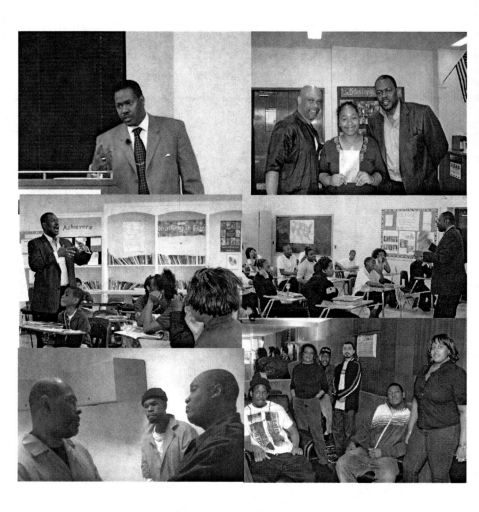

Facilitating a training in Chicago. My friend Walter of 30 years, helping me out at a career day school session. Speaking at Drew Freeman, and Thurgood Marshall. On the set of movie Reputations Fade Away with Ray Allen & Cliff Corry. In the studio recording my CD "Around the Mic w/Sir Charles & Friends" with Studio Engineer Filthy Rich, Jean Durr, Roop the Mastermind, Del "Sam Holla" McFadden, & his wife, my neice, Ms. Nikki aka Darlin Nikki McFadden.

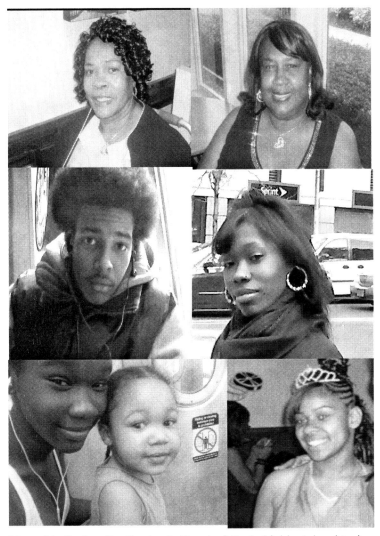

Mom, Big Sis Cecelia, Charles Jr.(Cee-Jay),Kychel (oldest daughter), granddaughters Destiny & Megan, Sasha Divine (youngest daughter)

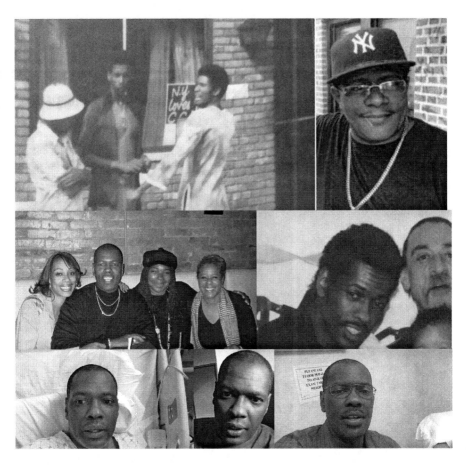

My brother Kyleke on the far right.
Diamond Dave R.I.P. I'll always love you primo (my cousin).
My sister Monique, my sweetie Sharon, my cousin Medina.
Picture of me and Pete back in the day when I was heavy on drugs.
2011 -2012 pictures of me fighting back the Lymphoma

Trueality Enterprises

Chapter 20

BIG FIGHT

Let me talk about the fights that I have had. There was second grade when I tried to be bold and bully a couple of kids. That was a fifty/fifty experience. One kid I caught in the hallway before class started. I nudged him and he nudged back letting me know that he was not scared of me. He was from out of town. I thought it would be a way to get my props and establishing myself as a straight up neighborhood bad boy. We tussled and he would not give in, that scared me. It was supposed to be easy. I had to learn boundaries. I think his name was Jeffrey Bradley, and we were around seven or eight years old.

The influence of our environment, other kids, and all sorts of things will either make you or break you. The lesson learned from that experience was to simply be who you really are. My brother may have been a bad boy, but I clearly was not and I was way out of line. I was trying to prove something to myself. This was the early 60's and martial arts were blossoming all over the country, mainly because of Bruce Lee and the Green Hornet, and I loved it. Now, I am not the tough type and I know I was not meant to be the tough type, but I was very young and I just kept pushing boundaries. I continued off and on trying to be the bold and brazen type.

My brothers were the types to fight and talk trash winning convincingly at it. I, on the other hand, had to find out who I really was. I had skills, but those were not at the top of my list. I was in my eighth grade gym class not having such a good day and one of the school bullies said something to me. I just simply said," *Your Mother.* "I was tired of him. Actually, I was not starting trouble this time, but I was fed up with him and his type. I just crossed the line and said the forbidden *your mother* comment. He threw his hands up and it was on. He started throwing punches and I started blocking and dodging. I didn't realize what I talked myself into. It all happened so quickly.

He grazed me with a punch to the face; but I tried to dodge it…as I was getting grazed, I was moving my head backward trying to avoid the punch. I jerked my head so fast backwards I banged my head right into a concrete wall. All I heard was a big ole empty sounding clunk-and I was knocked out for all of three seconds. I just stood there with my guard up unsure of what to do. Finally, it was broke up. There was no detention or suspension, the gym teacher just sent us on our way. The fight lasted for about ten minutes. That was another eye opening experience for me. OK, so I learned something from that experience. I was not a tough guy.

The pain of defeat was greater than anything I had ever experienced. It was also greater than anything I had ever hoped to experience in this lifetime. I was totally disgusted with myself, because after getting my kids enrolled in school and doing all

of the things a new parent is excited about; I allowed my drug use

to become the priority in my life and rob my children of their

father and a quality rearing from a paternal perspective.

I would tell my kids that I am going to read them a

story…I'd go buy some drugs and sneak back into the house, sneak

into the bathroom and just spend hours smoking crack. If I had

twenty dollars…it would not be enough to satisfy me. I would have

to sell one of my movies, a CD or something, so that I could

continue getting high. I would just make the kids wait. When I did

spend time with them, it was usually hurried. I would tell them I

am going to take them outside to play; I would rush through many

of the events that they wanted to participate in because finding

money to get high was more important. My relationship with their

mother dissolved over the years that we were together. She did

plenty of wrong too, but I was the main culprit that destroyed our

family.

My kids' mother told me many years before the children

were born about an old boyfriend ruined her life by taking money

from her for drugs. She said he was this big intimidating guy to

her. I remember thinking to myself that it was ridiculous and I am

not him. I never thought in my wildest imagination that I would

repeat the same pattern with her. I felt really bad about that aspect

of our relationship, because even if she was the worst person in the world nobody deserves to be taken advantage of especially to

the degree that a crack head will take you to.

Through my drugging, I took advantage of her. The

morning I woke up knowing I was finished with drugs was so

special that I will never forget it. In fact, I probably need to thank

my children for the guilt I felt. I love them so very much and it was

because of them that I couldn't stand getting high anymore. They

rescued me with their innocence, or as I say in my speeches "God

convicted me through the eyes of my children." I have not been

high since that day. It has been eighteen years. This is a fight that I

am still fighting, but for now I thank God I am winning big time.

The next fight was accepting and forgiving all of my

wrongdoing. It has been so hard, because my family is about

family and I destroyed the largest family opportunity that any man

would love to experience. I denied myself the opportunity to raise

my children. It is not the same when you raise or try to raise your

children from a distance. When they are on vacation in the summer

or when they visit on special occasions is hardly the approach to be

proud about. It may beat a blank, but it is still not the same.

So many fathers get a bad rap, and I must admit some of us

deserve the rap we are branded with. The truth is that it does not

matter whether it is for a season, because of a freak accident, or

even if nobody taught us better the bottom line is that you have

messed up. I have a simple theory when it comes to these

scenarios, and that is to just admit when you are wrong. Own up to it, your accuser loses power, and you keep yourself from making excuses about it.

Now there are a lot of us that either have changed our ways or simply never had an issue with ourselves, but maybe there was an issue with the child's mother. The number of dad's or fathers doing the right thing does not seem to compare to the dad's doing the wrong thing. However, you can't blame all of them for the actions of some of them. That will never fly as far as I am concerned. Give fathers credit for being fathers and at least making the effort to make the grade. I have to remember to always keep gratitude in my attitude. Today I do have my kids in my life, and they all seem to love me. That's a big success!

After being clean for several years my addictive behavior clung on to smoking cigarettes. As I began drug treatment we were given an allowance of cigarettes. I got hooked on the cigarettes instead of the reefer or the cocaine. It's been six or seven years that I have quit smoking cigarettes. I would like to think once again…I am winning this fight. What are the odds? I do not care about the odds; I just have to win this life battle.

I have put myself through so much. My mind is like that of a gladiator. I have to fight. I was this introverted kid, so unsure, so afraid of rejection, so out of place, so desperate to find myself in this big world. God allowed me to make so many mistakes, and I know he was with me every step of the way. This book is definitely for the reader that needs encouragement to know that it can be done, the reader that needs to know you are not the only one. I pray my spirit and philosophy find you as you read each word. Please, I beg you; allow my words and experience to be as vivid to you as the words on this paper. It is real, its Trueality!

My next fight is with the Big "C", Cancer. In or around 2000 I was diagnosed with Non-Hodgkin's Lymphoma. I do not totally buy into the fear aspect because I know how I feel and I know that God has a job for me. I have said that for a few years, but it is time for intervention now. I promise to give back and that is what I am going to do. I do think that God may be trying to get my attention. My cousin called me and asked me if I was interested in making some extra money, of course I was. Next, I wanted to know what I had to do. He told me I could help him out by being a mentor. I said yes and joined his team. I figured since I was a certified counselor and I was just beginning to take interest in being a Toastmaster, this would all be a plus in my experience. In the process of getting my paperwork together so that I could start working it was required to get an x-ray and when I did the doctors found an abnormality. Upon finding it, I had to follow up with my primary physician and he sang me the doom and gloom song.

God has empowered man to do some phenomenal things in this world, but I put my faith in God over man anytime. When I went home to tell my wife of the doctor's findings she didn't believe me. I am not only known as the upbeat positive one, but I am also known as the joker. I love to have fun She swore up and down that I was playing and she actually thought that I was carrying on my prank to long. When it finally hit her that I was serious, I knew that I had to be strong. I had to be strong not only for myself, but I had to be strong for the family also. I decided on a second opinion and went to Johns Hopkins in Baltimore. The doctors were amazed that I was not suffering any symptoms. They went down a checklist and it seemed as if nothing they asked me was affecting me. Finally, they asked me what I wanted to do and I told them nothing.

The decision had been made to do what they called wait and watch. Two to three years later I spoke to my oncologist and he informed me that the cancer spread to my back, hip, bicep, shoulder and it was still in my chest. The doctor gave me two years to live and I told him directly that his timetable has no effect on me; I simply will not accept that for my life, but it is time to take action. There is a book that says *faith without works is dead*, so I took action. This very well could be one of the biggest fights of my life, but I thank God that I have got the strength and the mind to fight it. They said that I need six months of chemotherapy, so let's get it on.

At the time my wife would make sure that I would make my appointments and she did what she thought I needed. I am not one for a lot of pampering or babying. That is just not my style and I do not respond to it well. I think my feeling is if I succumb to that type of treatment that I would not do things for myself and will rely on others. That is a sign of weakness in my eyes. I just felt like at that point in my life it was important that I must remain strong.

I never experienced a day of pain, before during or after treatment. I took the treatment for six months and everything seemed fine. I have done the before and after CAT Scans so that they can make comparisons with the diminished size of the growth. I am comfortable with that. I do not have much choice. It is at this point that I am proud to say that the Cancer as the doctor's see it is gone. I believe that you have to have faith in God, and in yourself. You do not have to be perfect about everything, but it is important to be grounded enough to know yourself. I have had many people praying for me and wishing well for me. I know that God has a plan for me. He wanted my attention, and he got it. Now I have got to do my part and keep my word to him. This book is just a small part of my job.

Life has changed for the better, but I still have debts and challenges. My life will not be above anyone else's life, but I have peace of mind now and I can appreciate why. I speak to people daily, sometimes I talk to co-workers and sometimes total strangers, but I try to encourage people everywhere I go I have been told that my daily email messages that I send have been read as far as Asia, and those people really appreciated the electronic encouragement. That fills my spirit.

Chapter 21

REMATCH

Well, it seems that the fight continues. Out of the clear blue sky I found myself in the hospital almost eleven years later. I was doing what I always do video production, music production, and working on trying to get a speaking engagement when my stomach started hurting me. At times it was hurting really badly, but I blew it off as a food consumption overload issue.

November 2011, I was experiencing these pains and discomfort, so I got a phone call from the benefits coordinator advising me to change my health package at work. Wondering what is going on, she goes on to explain to me that the state of New Jersey wanted to be sure that there was adequate health coverage for children and that they should be covered until age twenty-six. At the time I was covered with Kaiser Permanent and that was not enough because it was local coverage and not national coverage.

I decided to go with a new health provider Universal Life (GEHA) and needed to choose a doctor. Once that was out of the way I met with my new doctor, and began to tell him about my stomach pains and it was slowly getting worse. He referred me to a specialist and after two weeks of waiting, I got a phone call from my doctor advising me to go to the hospital immediately! I was thinking to myself how serious can it be? C'mon man, I am about to go to the movies. I am just saying that is where I was mentally because I didn't see anything like this coming.

The doctor told me that the diagnosis was that I had Jaundice. Reluctantly, I went to the Internet and looked up the best hospitals that handle Cancer and John's Hopkins and Georgetown University were at the top of the list. Georgetown was close and I decided that is where I would go. They took me into emergency, kept me all day, and then asked me to come back.

I must have been in the hospital off and on initially for about a month and I hated it. I hated every day that I was there because I was thinking about my job and my projects that I was setting up. If you know anything about me, then you know that I am always working on a project of some sort. Due to the fact that I have produced a lot of music, and some of it was really good I figured that I would produce another CD. This time it would be all about music, no poetry or anything else. I had not sung in quite some time, so that was another motivator for me. I was planning on making my last music CD as an artist; I would choose what I felt were my best songs and I would put them out.

I stayed in ICU for a few days and then they released me. It was beginning to become clear to me that this was a serious illness that I was addressing. Now you can call me crazy or stupid, but I was not afraid. I do have faith and this time around, this second life-threatening episode got me to thinking about what I could or should do.

I decided to video document my experience with the hopes that it could help someone else. Men are usually too bold, too stupid, or too something, but we do not take our health serious enough. I caught wind of the fact that people were seeing my video documentary and that they were really touched by it. I was grateful that I attempted to do something that did reach people.

The idea began to evolve. Finish your book and create another DVD to thank everybody that gave and showed support. That way I could create a product that was focused on a cause. Once I made up my mind to create the package it dawned on me to add the CD to the mix, so hence I have a CD, DVD, & book package.

Meanwhile, I still needed to get a PET scan, a Bone Marrow extraction, have a stint put in me so that the infection could pass through my pancreas and liver area, and of course I had to get chemo treatments. Getting back and forth to the hospital to make all of the appointments was shared by my family. A few times it would be my sister, but my girlfriend Sharon would make sure that I got to the majority of my treatments and appointments.

Relationships can be stressed because of illness, but I was fortune that Sharon was caring enough to take me without hesitation. One day she simply cried because of all that I had to go through and how she felt about me. If you saw the video on *you tube*, she is in the video for a quick moment when my daughter Kychel came up to see me from New York.

It was truly a surprise that my daughter came to see me.
She told me that she was going to come up but I didn't expect it. I
am learning that she is very concerned about my well-being. My
daughter and I got so close after she gave birth to my first
grandchild. There have been times when we would get on the
phone and just talk for hours. I am talking like two, three hours and
it is the same thing I do with my mother. I can talk to Mom about
any subject from A to Z for hours on end.

It is a great feeling to know that my children have that deep
a concern for my health. It is not something that I gave a lot of
thought to, but now that I know it, it sure warms my heart. I love
all of my kids like that. Thank God for our relationship.

The level of discomfort was crazy. I was itching all over
and scratching like a mad man. In my sleep, while awake, it
seemed like every moment of the day I was scratching. Eventually,
I went to a dermatologist and they did a biopsy and prescribed
some creams and ointments. There were ointments for my scalp,
my hands, and my body. I was so in tuned with my body.

My eyes were open for several reasons, and one was
because of the people that died while I was going through my
ordeal. A work colleague's daughter that was fifteen or so years
younger than me died of a brain tumor that was related to cancer of
some sort. She left a child behind. Her father is like a gentle giant.
He is a very nice guy and my heart felt for him. Another work
colleague was in the same hospital that I was in and I had the

opportunity to meet his wife and family. About a month later, his wife died.

Even when I returned to work, people seemed to be dying that I just didn't expect to die. My younger sister lost a friend that she knew for twenty years and it caused her to call me, because she knew what I went through. My life had been spared for a reason and I feel that reason is to be an inspiration and an encourager to all those that know me, know of me, or more importantly those that need to know what God can do in their life I was spared because there are things inside of me that I have not used, tapped into, or shared. We all have these gifts and it does matter whether we use them or not.

It is no longer about you when you realize you have a gift and you have been blessed. These two things are not one in the same. Many of us have been blessed, thank God for grateful blessings but it is the gift part that lays responsibility on your life. While receiving my chemo treatment twice a month I watched doctors, nurses, technicians and specialist do their jobs. Many are better than others, but they still have the same responsibility as the others..

Well to wrap this up, the bottom line for me is that I have to take the rest of life serious, but still enjoy it. I want to get back to basics. I have got a Health Master, endorsed by Montel Williams, so I juice at least twice daily. My diet consist of green veggies, some of the others also, fruits (apples, bananas, oranges blueberries, carrots, the whole healthy enchilada, plus Mondo water).

Now I still eat solids, but no fast food, hardly any greasy or fried food. When I made this change I was thinking about my kids. I hope they get finish with all of their foolish living, so they can prepare themselves for the possibility that life may want to throw them a curve ball. You just never know, so you have to be ready.

I saw a two hour video about a doctor named Stanislaw Brudzinski. Dr. Brudzinski is Polish, and has a practice in Texas. The thing about Dr. Brudzinski is that he is said to have a cure for cancer, but he is met with government opposition regarding his findings and his practice. The FDA, ACS, AMA have all seemingly made his life a living hell. According to the documentary there have been numerous patients that have and are willing to testify on his behalf to what he has done to cure their cancer, or their family member's cancer.

The doctor has been hauled into court numerous times but to no avail. His records have been confiscated; his documents have been copied and held on to for longer periods of time intentionally to disrupt his business. Anytime there has been a write up on the subject matter that Dr. Brudzinski has expertise in, his name has been clearly left out except on occasion when the may put his name on one line out of an entire document consisting of two pages or more.

If you were to come up with a cure for cancer, accidently or otherwise you can be arrested and incarcerated on the strength of the fact that the FDA, ACS, AMA and others control laws that determine how things are handled in the medical community. The bottom line is that sickness of all kinds is big business. If you interrupt that flow or that business you and I must be stopped at all costs.

That is exactly why alternative methods of treatment are scarce, and that is why our medical coverage can't be used for those scarcely available alternative options. If they should find that people are being cured, or finding that people have preference to alternative methods of treatment that is a no-no.

How greedy and evil can an individual or organization be? Evil and greedy enough apparently to not care about the Hippocratic Oath that was taken when they got into the profession of caring for the sick. I have recently met doctors who are ashamed of the treatment options Americans have because they know that it serves no curing purpose.

I went on to further my research by watching and reading up on a guy by the name of Michael Anderson. If you have ever heard of the Rave Diet, that is great! You know what I am talking about and where I am coming from. If you have not heard of the Rave Diet, then go to my site and follow the link to the product page www.Trueality.net and educate yourself. This is no joke;

people are dying because of lack of education, greed, and propaganda!

Despite your cultural belief system, the bottom line is we didn't always have modern technology invading our food supply now everything is big business. I understand about refrigeration, and keeping the food from going bad for health reasons. It is just we are out doing each other and ourselves so quick, so much, so often that it's shameful. That very shame is feeding into the decline of our welfare, and our morality. The bottom line is that big companies and agencies are taking advantage of us on multiple fronts and the health & wellness is one of those areas of focus.

We need to go back to nature or as Dr. Kloss said with the title of his book, *Back to Eden*. After I watched the two documentaries which took two different approaches on addressing cancer, diabetes, and all ailments, it hurt and angered me to find out the United States of America, would turn its back in favor of a buck, which we are supposed to have so many of anyway .

I understand that everyone will not be saved because of various variables. Some will just be too far-gone. Some will not know what is going on inside their bodies. I get it, some things are obviously impossible to stop, save, or change. However, for those that we can do something about, it should be done with the right intention in mind.

Chapter 22

COURAGE FACING MORTALITY

Confronting your demons or shortcomings is huge. It can be so difficult for us to look at ourselves and admit that we are not good at something or irresponsible. However, I am willing to gamble that is the difference maker when it comes to our growth and our evolution. At this stage of my life I frequently use the phrase: OPEN – HONEST – DIRECT. The reason is because I realize how difficult or uncomfortable it might be to communicate a particular thought, feeling, or idea. Therefore, if we are open, honest, or direct about what we are conveying, it will be picked up a lot better and reduces the gray area in communication. The communication we have with others is important, but so is the communication we have with ourselves.

This section is intended to give you a summary, or a bottom line for all of the junk that I have experienced. I told you all about what I did, who I did it with, and how I did it. Now I would like to primarily focus on the lessons that were learned or the main point about these various aspects. As I stated in the beginning of this book, this has been an almost twenty year project. Now that I have found purpose in re-visiting it I will complete it. As I observe my mentality throughout the various steps in the process I can see that my focus has changed. Initially I wanted it to be raw, because I am not ashamed of exposing the truth about my lack of tack, or my

lack of education when it comes to certain facets of my life.

I dare to say I have grown a little wiser through this

journey. Whoever knows me or takes a chance on this book could

have easily read about all sorts of garbage over the Internet instead.

Therefore, there is no need for me to spew anger, and needless

fornication to the reader. Stephen Covey passed away and one of

his many catch phrases referred to trying to leave the world a better

place before you die. With that being said, I will allude to the fact

that this is one of my ways in doing just that.

I was going to talk about every person and everything that I

had clashed with or interacted with. I had planned to discuss

everything that I did wrong along with everything that I learned,

and then it hit me why, who cares. I thought it was important, and

in many ways it actually is but I realize that there should be a more

honest purpose. If everything before this point was an appetizer

and an entrée, then this portion of the book has to be dessert.

My life's experiences have helped mold me into the person

I am today. I have learned that I still have to keep my mind open, I

have to share, and I also have to be willing to except. You have to

be willing to keep your mind open to life's lessons good or bad

simply because when you are open to these experiences you should

be able to learn from them. If it is a good experience then you

know how to enhance your situation the next time you encounter

the same circumstances and if it is negative you know what not to do again or what to look out for. The sharing aspects are equally important because nobody knows everything.

By sharing, you show that you are not afraid to deal with your own experiences good or bad and you position yourself to learn from others. You may get knowledge on things that you never considered. That knowledge can be the difference between doing and not doing, growing or just being stagnant. You will also learn from someone's experience and avoid a lot of pain.

Acceptance is so important because we learn in life that sometimes we are powerless over the things that happen. When you are powerless, acceptance is probably the best thing in my opinion. We can still learn from it, but we do not have to stress over those things because we can't control or dictate the outcome. It does not matter how you feel, if you do not have the power to change your situation, grow from it and move on.

What I have learned from many of my mistakes was that they brought me to where I am today. When I tie that into my ministry, my sense of purpose or my calling is something that I can give back to the world. When I would manipulate, steal, or con people for money, it was for purely for my own self-indulgent purposes. Selling personal valuables was for personal gain also. I can take those same ways and use them for good today.

Instead of talking people out of something, I can talk them into seeing something within, helping them to recognize their own personal talents or abilities or show them ways to recognize the talent and abilities of others. Instead of selling valuables for drugs, I can sell books, CDs, tools, and tips to educate people on drug life and for their personal development. Bad habits and bad ways can be transformed into positive energy and purposes. Hopefully we are still growing in the process and discovering new ways to achieve this. I have been told that you can't keep it if you are not willing to give it away, so I will be giving away my life's lessons at every opportunity afforded to me.

It is so important that I survive and persevere to do great things. I have seen so much and I have met so many people that have fallen to ways of the world. Others have gone on to do well for themselves, but we are all flesh and blood. Almost all of my life I have lived in my head listening to the inner voice. Many times I didn't know what I was listening to, but now four decades later I know exactly what it is. Dear God I beg and plead maybe even with a little more help than you usually give to me I pray that you put your blessing on me Lord. I want so badly to matter more than a little bit. I am human yet alien to what the inevitable has in store for me. I shall constantly fight for more.

I have written several times; and it's true God has a plan for my life, so I have got to finish this project and share with as many people as possible. Show our young people how to be aware of the pitfalls of life and how not to become a statistic. Folks we have got to clear the hurdles and obstacles of life! You can be an overcomer! We can't take anything with us when we die. Do an inventory, what has this drug addict accomplished after the mess I created? I gave my life to God first and foremost. I have been able to re-establish my relationship with my children I have become a Federal Employee where I have trained law enforcement officers of the Federal Reserve. I am a former president of a Toastmaster's club (ATM-B, CL), a public speaker (former NSA member), a certified biblical counselor, a mentor, a singer and a lyricist, an author, cinematographer, a videographer, an editor, an actor...get the picture.

Now how many people do you know that are more talented than I am in one or more of these areas? I bet many of you are. Believe me if you are given the opportunity, you may surprise yourself. It is not about me, and has not been for a long time now; I just had to open my eyes to realize it. Usually in life, the lesson does not come until after the fall.

I have met and learned from some of the best minds in the world. I am talking about motivational speakers, business trainers, corporate leaders, politicians, no names, etc. (Les Brown, John C. Maxwell, Jim Rohn, T.D. Jakes, Pastor Patrick Walker of The New Macedonia BC and Pastor Rogers of Triumphant BC in the Hyattsville, MD, Pastor Rick Warren and Pastor Joel Osteen. The list of philosophers and role models include Muhammad Ali, Bruce Lee, and Anthony Browder). These are some of the most prominent minds that I have been grateful to experience. One man that will always be an inspiration to me is my brother whom I have not seen since I was a teenager, Anthony Lewis Smith aka

Kyleke Allah.

Two men that I really look up to are my former boss Billy

Sauls and Willie Jolley. Sauls was the Chief of the Federal

Reserve Law Enforcement. He has given me personal time and has

done things outside of what any boss should do. In my opinion he

is more like a big brother or father figure. That is not easy to say

about another man when you are already grown, but those are my

feelings. This man was supportive in allowing the mystique of Sir

Charles to remain alive, mainly as a motivational speaker and

trainer.

Willey Jolley has been my personal motivator and

conscious. I met him several times, and then I got to know him on

a personal level. When you look up to someone like a Willie Jolley

or a Les Brown, and they give you their personal cell phone

number or they meet you for lunch and they're not on the clock

how much better does it have to get? He gave me the keys to a

white Benz one day. Okay, I am just kidding about that I just want

to make sure you're still paying attention. He saw me before I saw

him and calls me out. "Sir Charles, what you are up to!" Yes the

small things can be priceless.

His story always struck a chord with me, the singer that

turned into a speaker and he can still chirp!

And you know what? I still have work to do on myself, and

I am still charged to give to others. I have been fortunate enough to have the opportunity to speak at so many forums. Given the opportunity to invigorate and educate young people on the wiles of a negative lifestyle has been a gift. Teaching Sunday school and Bible study is just a small, yet very important piece of the puzzle. I have been able to perform around the country, as well as outside of the country, and I consider myself extremely fortunate. I am able to give back and I want to.

After I turned my life around, it was important for me not to run from my people. I wanted to be sure that I learned from my past and that my treatment was not something that I got, but something that I lived. I moved to DC from New York as a married man, and a man on a mission. I always felt that I would live in the DC area again, but I didn't know when or how. I started looking for work as soon as the move was made. I was ready to learn how because in New York, you just did.

I looked in the newspaper and one of the companies I saw had a symbol that resembled a crucifix as their logo, or at least it looked like one to me. I answered the ad by faxing my resume, which was in my living room. Then I went to my bedroom and prayed a simple prayer. As I came out of my bedroom, the telephone was ringing; it was the agency asking me to come in for an interview. They had reviewed my resume and wanted to test me. I went into northwest DC the very next day, interviewed and scored well. I arrived home after the interview process; walked in the door and ten minutes later I received a phone call from the agency asking me to work a two-week assignment, answering phones for them.

We negotiated the rate, and I started the next day. I was a little uncomfortable after the first week because I liked the place and I only had a week left. At the end of my assignment, I asked the supervisor to call me back if they needed me, and she told me to come back on Monday. It turned into a long-term assignment. I stayed at that company for five or six months, interviewed for different departments, and eventually they made me an offer. I was so excited I couldn't believe it. Then an offer was made for me to work off sight. I loved it.

The point of the matter is that events like these do not just happen every single day. They can, but rarely do. That is why I believe in the power of prayer and I know that my life has been blessed. After having this job for three years, something else happened. The company, which was about eighty-nine years old and internationally known with about 85,000 employees, collapsed because of the actions of a few greedy souls.

My mindset was simply, next. There were other people there that were so upset and afraid because they didn't know what their future would be like and they didn't know about money that they had invested within the company. Many of my co-workers didn't understand why I was so calm in the midst of this situation. I have God in my life and I know that He would care for me, and I also know that when we are powerless over a situation we are powerless. I didn't have a stash or a nest egg to rely on. I applied for unemployment just like everybody else and I used the resources they offered us.

I was eventually asked to see one of the big bosses and he said he felt bad, but they would have to let me go. After I left his office, I feverishly sent out resumes, made appointments and walk-ins. I realized after about a week or so later that I had not prayed about it. So I stopped looking for work at that very moment and I prayed. I prayed a very specific prayer. It was summer and my kids were coming down to spend it with me. I asked the Lord to allow me to spend quality time with my kids, and that I would resume looking for work in the fall Believe it or not, that is exactly what happened, to the dollar. I was able to enjoy time with the kids, and a week before they were to go home, I received a call regarding a job. They gave me a start date. For me, that was further proof that God was there for me and He was looking out for me.

Is it a perfect life yet? I always say it is what it is, and what does that mean? Whatever happens there is no in between. Things do not happen the way they are supposed to happen for no reason at all. You have to have faith, you have to believe in yourself, you have to believe in God, you have to believe that God has a purpose for your life and you have to live like you believe it. You can't just say the words; you have to tell yourself that it is what it is.

Through this writing, I hope you can see how God has had his hand on my life. Through all the successes that I have shared, through all of the realization of whom I am and what I am capable of, He has been there every step of the way. He has had his hand on my life, been a part of my life, all my life and it took me thirty plus years to figure it out. That is Courage Facing Mortality

Chapter 23
A PERFECT LIFE

I look back over these pages, and I find that a good book does not have to be long and neither does life. I know most of us would prefer a long life. How many times have you said you wished the book, the movie, the story didn't end like this or that...they should have...or all they needed to do is? Yeah, me too, I've done it countless times. This brings me to another question. Is a perfect life long or short? Does life have to be perfect...can it be?

My experiences say so many different things: music, love, sex, drugs, jobs, lifestyle, choices, and the list go on. There's one common denominator—God—that I never realized was always there. My life-changing experiences tell me that I am just a regular man from the inner city like many others, and I had questions about whom, what and why. When I stopped questioning so much and went out into the world and started living, I received a lot of the answers. Yet my life's experiences would eventually tell me that I am not like everybody else, and that I do not have to be.

The Six, or the ear-to-ear principle, relates to the True-alities of life. We have the truth and reality, everything else speaks for itself. Most people follow traditional methods of living, adapting to what the masses do, others are a little torn between conventional methods and being their own person, and finally you have the total, out-of-the-box persona. That out-of-the-box persona is usually viewed as a loner, a troublemaker, or as the something's- wrong-with-them type.

That same mindset is needed when being innovative or creating, a wave that has never been seen before. I encourage all people to be their authentic true self. Nobody has to put handcuffs on you, or lock you away in a traditional jail cell in order for you to be enslaved. The way you think and decide to do things is what determines whether you are truly free. If you say it, then mean it and stand beside it claim it! Only because of God's purpose for my life have I been able to overcome the old lifestyle. After using acid, angel dust, and everything else that I've mentioned, I am blessed to have a functioning brain, as well as reasonable health. Yes, even though I had to deal with Cancer.

That takes me to an entirely different level. I did so many drugs in my life that if my limbs and organs had mouths, they would probably scream "STOP! STOP!" I am very fortunate that I was diagnosed with Non-Hodgkin's Lymphoma a few years ago. I do not know the stats, but I do know that many people have complications from chemotherapy. Either their hair falls out or they get sick to the stomach. I never experienced those things. Maybe a little nausea, but that was it. Some people would say that it is in remission, but the way I see it, it is gone. Even before the chemo, I never suffered any particular symptoms or discomfort. The only thing I experienced was fatigue. So what is a perfect life? Is it literally carefree from worries, perfect health, financially stable or excessive wealth? What good is it to have those things if you have nobody to share it with or nobody that you can pass it on to? Thankfully, God has a plan for my life and that plan is to give and do.

I mentored a young man from DC, and after I stopped mentoring him, he was murdered a month later. It was very upsetting to my family because the young man spent time with us. He ate dinner with us, went to the movies with my sons and I, played video games with us and after a while we got attached. It was very awkward to see him lying in a casket at sixteen years old. After that incident, I have continued to try to give back. I spoke at a high school in Maryland where I met two teenagers—a young man and a young lady—who were to graduate. They seemed to be very well behaved, down to earth kids with a sense of focus. They got jobs through an internship at my company. A woman from my church set it up for them.

It continues to amaze me how God places people in your life. After his high school graduation, this same young man was presented with the opportunity to mentor a junior high school kid. My young friend is in college, but we sat down and discussed mentoring, and again, it amazes me how life repeats certain cycles. I mentored someone personally, and through my ability to reach people, a young man I reached is mentoring someone also. It is called *paying it forward*. It made me feel really good to know that he is doing something that I have done and I hope he can reach the

kid and make a difference while he gains something from the
experience. This is the ultimate reward. Someone that has looked
up to me now has someone looking up to him. A generation of
positive influence is a success. I am fortunate that I have been able
to witness this success in my lifetime. It is sort of like giving birth
and watching your child grow up to become a successful
businessperson or invent something that saves lives…what a great
feeling.

This is another reason why I feel the constant need to have
God in my life. His blessings can flow through us all. When I am
feeling down, it is good to know that I have touched someone.
When I look into one of their faces, receive an e-mail or phone call
from one of them, I am lifted simply because it makes me feel
good to know that I have a personal connection that God has
arranged and there is no need for me to be down. That is so
important. "You can't keep it, if you are not willing to give it
away," is what I say often.

In Washington, DC, I attended The New Macedonia Baptist
Church. As a member, I grew, not because of the teaching or
counseling, because my spirit was fed and I learned about myself
and God. There are a few important things about Christian life that
are essential. We all want to have good favor in life. Since being a
member at The New Macedonia Baptist Church, Pastor Walker
talked about "Obeying God's Word" Jonah 1. This seems to be so
simple, but just like with a child, we learn and get good at things

through repetition and a desire to understand. If we all could get this one thing right, everything else would fall in place. I am still striving to obey. Pastor Walker talked about "How to Handle Temptation." Pastor Walker went into James 1, and he stressed the fact that we need to reflect on our purpose. If you do not know your purpose you better ask somebody, and not just anybody. We also need to trust in the Lord. Pastor Walker went on to talk about how evil thoughts lead to evil actions and how our test / temptations are tailor-made for each and every one of us, and this makes us very vulnerable. It is ultimately important that we develop a dynamic faith. There is so much to be said about each of these topics, but I feel deep in my heart that we need to keep it real; we need to be accountable and responsible for our choices. You do not really need someone to drill it in your head about everything that you do so often that is wrong. *If we are honest with ourselves, we know when we make wrong moves.* Through it all, we are human and we will make mistakes, but we can profit from our mistakes. Pastor Walker has assured us that we need to recognize our mistakes for what they are, and they are a trick of Satan. I am not a preacher, but if you really want to have a good life and are willing to fight the good fight, there is no telling what you can have. I hope these chapters make sense to you and inspire you to make change.

I remember how it was, before I found God, before I really found Him. I was the typical follower of foolish ways, foolish things, constantly trying to fit in. I viewed myself as a big time square, with an extremely high need of acceptance. Constantly feeling like an outsider, I eventually realized that it was not that important that I had to fit in with the fads of today; I had to have what everybody else had. As it stands today, I still do not have what everybody else has, and I do not want what everyone else has. I feel good just to be so different. It took me a few decades, but I got here. Many of us call ourselves Christians, but do not talk like one, look like one, and act like one. I do not have it going on, but I am aware when I mess up, and I honestly strive to correct my ways. And you know what else; I get that feeling of not being like everyone else every time I try to check myself. It's so easy to mess up versus doing the right thing. I remember how important I thought it was to fit in with cool kids or the older kids.

So today, it is okay for me to be corny because I remember not fitting in. I look forward to saying "Good morning" to people, encouraging someone, smiling at someone or trying to help when I can (I am still not 100%). Growing up, had someone smiled at me, encouraged me, patted me on the back, or told me it was going to be all right, who knows how things would have turned out. However, by the grace of God, there go I. Although things didn't work out perfectly for me, the Lord allowed me to make certain choices; He was still there (because He had a plan for my life). I just hope that someone can see the God in me, when I am smiling.

ABOUT THE AUTHOR

Charles Cary aka Sir Charles is a motivational speaker, and has been a certified customer service trainer since 2005, in addition he's a certified trainer from Homeland Security in Law Enforcement Instruction, also since 2005.

His achievements include being, a current member of Toastmaster's International (Past President of Toastmasters ATM-B, CL), a former silver certificate holder of the Life Insurance Millionaires Roundtable, and a former member of the National Speakers Association. He feels that many of these opportunities has prepared him to do the things that are most need in our society today. The giving, sharing, and teaching components in our communities are greatly needed. That's why he's also a founding member of MOST (American Mothers Maryland Chapter).

What he loves to do is work , and he's passionate about it. When it comes to singing, writing a song, filming, editing, facilitating training or giving a speech-that when he's at his best!

He loves engaging people more than anything. He's a DC native that considers New York City his true home and wouldn't have it any other way. A true entrepreneur, he loves adding value in all that he does. That is the principle thing for Charles.

Fun for Charles comes on various levels. His hobbies are watching movies, and playing video games. He has 3 children, and 2 grandchildren with one on the way.

SERVICES

Training Workshops and Keynote Speeches
Advertising Production and Editing
Music Production and Leasing

www.Trueality.net

www.Affordableads.net

CREDITS

PUBLICIST: Fran Briggs

PUBLICIST: Reba Barnes

EDITOR: TWA Solutions (Jessica Tilles)

Book Cover Concept: Charles Cary

Graphic Design: "A Splash of Moet" (Monique Medina)

Book Cover Photo: El Shamesh Photography (Enoch El Shamesh)

CD Cover Photo: Roberts Digital (Lenon Roberts)

DVD Cover Photo: Sky Media (Kwan Taylor)

CPSIA information can be obtained at www.ICGtesting.com
Printed in the USA
BVOW070109281112

306581BV00001B/3/P